Clear Skin

Clear Skin

✦

Organic Action Plan for Acne

A Safe, Step-by-Step, Individualized Guide to Clear Acne with Diet, Stress Relief, and Organic Skincare

Julie Gabriel

iUniverse, Inc.

New York Lincoln Shanghai

Clear Skin
Organic Action Plan for Acne

iUniverse books may be ordered through booksellers or by contacting:

iUniverse
2021 Pine Lake Road, Suite 100
Lincoln, NE 68512
www.iuniverse.com
1-800-Authors (1-800-288-4677)

ISBN-13: 978-0-595-42460-3 (pbk)
ISBN-13: 978-0-595-86794-3 (ebk)
ISBN-10: 0-595-42460-0 (pbk)
ISBN-10: 0-595-86794-4 (ebk)

Printed in the United States of America

To Mama, Vlad, Maria.

Contents

INTRODUCTION

"You have such a great skin," a skincare spokesperson told me while we were enjoying a low-carb organic lunch at some product presentation party. She said it casually, as if it was a matter of fact. I smiled and thanked her, of course, but my soul was in tears.

Fifteen years of scrubbing, toning, peeling, moisturizing, massaging, burning, freezing, acupuncturing, tanning and bleaching—and all I get is "great skin?" I deserve "fabulous, amazing, wonderful"—not less!

In panic I tried to remember what I applied to my skin that morning. Most likely, I used a potent mattifying makeup primer underneath an industrial-strength camouflage concealer for my pimples and acne spots. And then it hit me. I don't use concealers anymore. In fact, all I was wearing on my skin that day was a sunblock and some sheer mineral powder foundation.

Perhaps I finally did something right, if even skincare professionals comment on my complexion. I wish I've heard this when I was fifteen years younger. How much embarrassment, heartbreak, insecurity and money loss I would have avoided!

This is why you are reading this book. You too are tired of discomfort and shrinking self-esteem thanks to less-than-perfect skin. In the society that expects us to have perfect looks, clear healthy skin is vital for success as much as for your general well-being. Most likely, you can't wait till someone tells you how great you look today—with or without makeup!

Before I came up with this book I have read about forty different books and reports on skincare, not to mention thousands of articles in professional or glossy magazines. Besides, I am personally responsible for at least 500 published pieces on skincare, beauty and well-being.

And no matter how much we pay for information—5 dollars for a glossy magazine or twice as much for a book about beauty—there are two polar kinds of skincare knowledge we end up with: fast-food facts and quick tips in women's magazines reprinted every year (how many times have you been told to apply the bronzer on the apples of your cheeks?) or solid science-loaded tomes that require a thesaurus and a good deal of patience to read till the end.

I think that we all need something easy-to-understand and ready-to-use, a guide that we can make work for us immediately. This guide should be fun, too, because the moment we stop enjoying the skincare routine, it stops working. Have you ever noticed? We skip the toner if it smells bad, we are too busy to pack on masks if they are not funny-looking, strawberry-smelling, or bright blue, and we would rather use a loofah on our faces than exfoliate with a scrub that doesn't smell like vanilla latte.

We are women, we tend to surround ourselves with things that are pretty and sweet-smelling, and we all try to have fun when we take care of our skin—even when we battle our skin's worst invaders, pimples and wrinkles. And just as you read this, real women like you and me are pondering in the pharmacy skincare isle staring at bottles and tubes trying to find a working solution for their blemishes.

Beauty industry tosses out new products every month, and something that was so "in" and "hot" last month is history today. No matter how seductively looks that spa-worthy white tube with some medical mumbo jumbo on the box, general basics of healthy skin will never change. If the product in a pretty tube doesn't work today, it won't work tomorrow, even if they package it in a clear glass bottle with an elegant golden cap.

Whenever you notice a pimple, it's time to fight acne. Whenever you encounter itchy scratchy area it's time to pare down your beauty regimen and calm down your skin. Whenever you feel a bump ripening under skin surface, you need to treat it efficiently and gently to prevent dark spots and scars from happening.

While there is no 100% sure-proof cure for pimples, the only available strategy for us is prevention and consistent care so that the next outbreak doesn't happen in the first place.

Just like you cannot detoxify the skin from outside, you can't clear the skin disorder when it shows up on the skin surface. Whenever you have a skin allergy, you don't only try to calm the itching, you look for reasons that might've caused it, be it grapefruits or macadamia nut. Same is true when it comes to acne. When you see a pimple, it's not because your skin is bad, it's because something bad is happening inside. You should take a good look on what you put inside your body (fried food, sugar-laden drinks, and all those vanilla bean lattes), you should take a good look on your jitteriness and worries, and you should take a damn good look below your belly button. Your skin problems begin in your bowels, brains and ovaries. Whatever happens on the skin's surface, it's just an aftereffect.

The worst thing about problem skin is that it's totally unpredictable. If you have one single blemish, it means you can have more in future, when you least expect it. This book will help you clear your acne blemishes and avoid skin irritations in future.

Clear Skin: Organic Action Plan for Acne does not insist that you should buy certain skin care items to treat your skin blemishes. Neither does it promote any beauty brand nor a medication. This book appreciates the fact that all our skins are different, not only in color, but in their inner living mode. What works for a fair-skinned woman with blonde hair may never work for a teenager with a dark skin, and vice versa.

As a result, this book will provide you with the essential information you need to pick the skin care products that work for you, your own skin type, your age and gender. You should never treat your acne with the same products and procedures that are suitable for a teenager if you are well over 30. Products that are great for women may not work for men, because their skin is different. What works for a dark-skinned girl in her 20s will never be suitable for a professional woman in her 30s. Skincare routine that is fine with a teenager will damage an unborn baby inside a woman who is suffering a sudden acne outbreak during pregnancy.

These is why we take a look at different types of acne-prone skin and introduce not one but **six** different acne regimens: for teenagers, for young women with fair skin tones, for pregnant women and newborns, for dark-skinned women and men, for men in general, and for women in their menopause.

You are more than welcome to review all the segments, because you might find solutions or products that are compatible with your own skin concerns.

WHAT'S DIFFERENT ABOUT CLEAR SKIN: ORGANIC ACTION PLAN FOR ACNE

This is a practical, fun, and easy to use guide to achieving clear skin and battling acne, blemishes and post-acne scars.

Who needs this book?

This book is essential to anyone who suffers from blemishes, or acne, from occasional blemishes to full-blown acne attacks.

What makes this book unique?

Clear Skin: Organic Action Plan for Acne features plain-English explanations and newest research on acne plus customized treatment strategies that really make a difference.

Clear Skin: Organic Action Plan for Acne includes step-by-step skin care routines for every skin type affected by acne, from teenagers to pregnant women and women entering menopause.

Clear Skin: Organic Action Plan for Acne includes easy-to-grasp down-to-earth facts that you can use to achieve clear healthy skin right away.

First of all, you will get to know why acne happens and what causes your skin to erupt with pimples, whiteheads and blackheads. Why do you need it? You cannot fight something unless you really know its nature. You don't know why pimples pop up—neither doctors nor serious MD-bearing researchers do. Therefore, you don't know how to properly care for your particular type of problem skin, and even if I tell you how, you won't know why.

While many people generally understand what sebum is and why sugar is bad for skin, many still rely on brief catchy marketing pitch found on boxes with latest miracle potion. Many years of beauty reporting and research have convinced me that cosmetic industry doesn't want women to become their own skin experts. When women realize what actually works for their problem skin, they will stop falling prey for newest marketing tricks. As a result the multibillion dollar beauty industry which relies on our poor knowledge, fragility and lack of self-esteem will suffer significant losses.

Just think about it. How many times you spent $50 on a 'revolutionary' acne kit or even a single product that promised you clear skin and stashed it in your bathroom drawer because this product either dried up your skin so it peeled or broke you out even more? But your money is gone. Everyone from copywriter to chemist to brand manager and store clerk got paid.

This happens because you don't understand what exactly is going on with your skin. As a result you use wrong products, eat the wrong food, practice the wrong kind of fitness regimen, and spend more and more money on products that you are never going to use or that make you look even worse.

When it comes to acne, most people are still wandering in the dark, buying anything that gives them some hope, losing their money to talented marketers and gifted packaging designers.

To properly care for your acne-prone skin, you need a special routine that considers all the processes that lead to acne and is perfectly tailored to your skin color, ethnicity, age, sex and budget. This way, *you* control your acne, instead of letting acne control you, your life, your career and your relationships.

As a woman who was suffering from acne for years and was lucky to get her hands to the newest and latest in skincare and makeup, I personally tried all the beauty options mentioned in this book. Just like you, I battled my acne for years, until I calculated the most effective regimen for my skin type. However, when I recommended it to my olive-skin-toned girlfriend, she still had acne. Then I started to realize that if something cures acne in fair Caucasian skin doesn't necessarily benefit more dense Asian skin. I started digging deep in my books.

Soon I understood that my mother who developed acne in her 50s and a teenager next door who's battling his first pimples, they are all prescribed the same benzoyl peroxide lotions and potions. I was furious. My Mom's skin is thin, wrinkled and fragile after years of sunbathing and recent chemical peels. How dare they treat her the same way they treat a teenage boy with young and taut skin?

I can absolutely relate to your anguish and frustration caused by zits and pimples erupting just when you least expect them. I have many friends who were too busy or too shy to turn up at dermatologist's office with their red hot pimples and zits. Yet, they had to do something about it, so they hit the drugstore isles looking for the remedy.

Because each person with problem skin becomes prone to acne for his or her own reasons, not all acne skincare products will work for everyone. When I was trying to fight my own acne using conventional methods I was often astonished by totally contradicting marketing claims. I tried to work out a universal yet individualized skincare routine for people with different skin types who face acne. This way, we don't leave any skin factor overlooked, and that's why my recommendations really work for many absolutely different skin types.

With my skin type descriptions at the beginning of each chapter you will easily identify which regimen is better suited for you. With my suggestions in each chapter you can build your own skincare routine that works for your skin type, not against it. Based on your own sensations you will pick the products that are more or less fast-acting, maybe more or less expensive. None of the suggested acne skincare regimens is alike; 50-year-old pre-menopausal acne sufferer should not use the same products as a teenager coping with his first attack of zits. You know which age group you belong to; hence you won't have any problem identifying the right routine.

As a result, you won't need to buy every new acne product anymore. You will only use what your skin really needs and what really works for your skin. Your daily beauty regimen will be simple and cost-effective. Following the detailed skincare routine developed for your unique skin condition you will no longer be a slave to your acne blemishes and pimples because we will together work to prevent them from happening.

In the beginning of this book we will introduce you to the basics of the human skin and will explain why the mere construction of the skin makes acne so easy to happen. Then we will discuss what acne really is, and why it is not a skin disorder but rather an inflammatory disease that results from many bodily functions and malfunctions. You will understand how diet and emotions affect acne and what you can do to prevent acne from happening. This is a universal segment that appeals to any age group, sex or ethnicity. For many of you this would be the most important segment of the book—and believe it or not, by simply altering you lifestyle choices you can greatly diminish your acne.

Once you become familiar with acne and your own skin, we will provide each and every acne sufferer with complete skincare regimen that would tame existing acne blemishes, help erase acne marks and scars and prevent future acne outbreaks. Teens, pregnant women, men, women approaching menopause and women in their 20s and 30s, people with darker skins and people with lightest skin who suffer from acne and dry skin, all of these categories of acne sufferers will find an appropriate acne solution for their specific skin type.

This book focuses on natural approaches to problem skin, and most of the products mentioned in the specific chapters are either organic, which means they were created without toxic chemicals from plants grown in strict accordance with international organic guidelines without the use of pesticides, or contain minimal possible chemical additives. I will explain why preservatives, penetration enhancers, emollients, fragrances and other chemical fillers found in skincare today actually work against your skin and exacerbate your acne instead of healing it.

Each of these skin-specific chapters contains detailed daily skincare plan along with recommendations of natural skincare products suitable for your skin condition and lifestyle. To succeed in achieving clear skin it is important to be consistent and follow these recommendations precisely. I will provide you with step-by-step plans to fight acne and remove acne spots and marks, as well as suggestions on maintenance of clear skin you will end up with. You will find products that work best for your skin condition along with suggestions on how to fit them into your budget. This way, you will buy only products that you need instead of wasting money on all the new lotions and potions that hit the market. You will learn the best way to cleanse your skin, to use toners, to shave without pain and irritation, to smooth wrinkles while keeping acne at bay. I will offer you many choices so that you can find the right organic product that fits your budget and is available in your area. I will recommend which products will help you stay acne-free, such as post-shave balms for men, anti-wrinkle and anti-acne products for women over 40, mattifying oil-free moisturizers for young acne sufferers. I will also provide you with the list of beneficial ingredients that may be helpful for your specific skin concerns so you could expand your beauty knowledge and look out for new natural products that we may not know yet about. In addition to that you will find supplemental and nutritional suggestions that will complement your specific age and lifestyle group.

For every skin category we will provide some additional anti-acne and scar procedures that will help you in your acne battle if you find that non-prescription medications are not really effective. Before you try any advanced acne treatment we recommend that you consult with your dermatologist or family doctor. I will offer some specific advice on prescription-only medications and procedures so that you are ready for your appointment—I know acne is a sensitive issue, and we want you to be as much informed as possible. Please note that I will *never ever* ask you not to visit dermatologist and read this book instead.

UNDERSTAND YOUR SKIN

Glowing flawless skin is a dream of all women. Smooth skin represents beauty, sexual attractiveness and self-confidence. Unfortunately, acne turns skin into opposite of smoothness. Red swollen bumps, pus and black dots are ugly on their own, and they are usually followed by unsightly scars and spots that are equally hard to eliminate.

Skin is the largest organ in the human body. Skin makes up about 15% of our total weight and covers 20 square feet on an average person. Even wrinkled, bruised or age-spotted, skin still protects us from the environment, inhales oxygen, safely cushions our inner organs, feels and sends to the brain all the sensations from the outside world, cools our body systems, eliminates waste and toxins. As if all that wasn't enough, skin makes us beautiful and unique! That's why we must keep our skin healthy so that it can glow with beauty and perform its vitally important tasks.

A mechanism more complex than any computer in the world, skin can perfectly repair itself. In fact, it's the only organ that can completely restore itself when damaged. All the scratches, cuts, wounds, or burns heal eventually and most often without a sign.

If you suffered a cut, take a look at how fine yet firm skin is at the place of the opening. You will never see a fabric so reliable as skin!

ANATOMY OF THE SKIN

Skin Layers

To understand what happens with your skin when you have acne, you need to know something of the way skin works, so to start I will describe in a few words how skin is made up.

Let's begin with the top layer, ***stratum corneum***, is formed of 25-30 layers of dead layered flattened skin cells that are rich in keratin. Stratum corneum protects the skin and continually renews itself by flaking off dead skin and replacing it with newer cells. On most parts of the skin the top dead skin cells layer is very thin, only 0.15 mm deep, and on the palms and soles of the feet this layer is much thicker—about 0.5 mm.

Underneath the stratum cornea is an epidermis, the living top portion of the skin, and a **basal membrane**, which works as a communicator between two most important skin layers. What we need to know is that acne scarring happens when the basal membrane is broken by acne widespread. To avoid damaging this layer, you must treat acne as soon as possible.

Under the epidermis is a **dermis,** or **basal layer.** This is the very busy skin layer that delivers nourishment and protective skin cells to epidermis layer. Dermis layer is formed of collagen and elastin molecules, two proteins that provide the skin with the density and flexibility. Dermis also contains blood vessels, as much as 19 yards of blood vessels per square inch, plus nerve endings. They reach right up to the base of the epidermis but don't actually penetrate it. When people have pimples, or inflamed acne lesions, most of the inflammation take place in the dermis, which results in scarring.

The **subcutaneous layer** is the deepest layer of the skin. It is built of lipocytes, or fatty cells, that work as energy storage and a buffer for the enormous blood pressure that our skin holds from within. The subcutaneous layer is the skin factory. There your body manufactures new skin cells. As the skin cells are produced they migrate upward through the three middle layers of the epidermis. As they do, they get farther and farther away from the blood and nutrients they need to survive. By the time they reach the outside world they are dead. There is nothing left for them to do but flake off so the next batch of cells can arrive.

As skin cells grow and mature, they move up to the stratum cornea, become dry and flat, eventually shedding off. This process is called desquamation. It takes, on average, about twenty-eight days for a skin cell to travel from the base of the epidermis to become a dry keratinized cell at the top of the epidermis and then be shed at the surface of the stratum cornea layer. When your skin becomes oily, these dead cells stick to excess sebum and form a paste that clogs pores.

When we age, skin cells turnover slows by 50 per cent, which shows up as wrinkles and rough skin surface. One inch of skin is formed by 9,500,000 cells, so dead cells even being scrubbed off by, say, glycolic peels, do not pose any danger to the consistency of the skin.

Pores

Sit in front of the mirror and gently pull the skin on your face. You will see lots of tiny dots, pink or black craters that may be empty and clean or filled with black substance. A pore consists of a highly coiled secretory portion deep in the dermis, which forms a tiny bulb, and a relatively straight duct conducts the secretions toward the surface of the epidermis.

Pore is a tiny duct in the skin, called a ***follicle***. If you look at the pore structure, it will look like a rabbit's hole in the skin. There are two kinds of pore on your face: the openings with hair follicles in them and tiny openings to sweat glands. It is important to understand the difference between two kinds of pores because sweat glands and sweat production are not directly linked to acne. That is why you cannot cleanse pores and remove acne-causing blockages ("impurities" or "toxins") either by steaming in a spa, visiting a sauna or vigorous exercise in the gym. The sweat is made by a different gland and emerges onto the skin through a completely different pore.

Another type of pores contains a sebaceous (oil) follicle and sometimes a hair. Inside this "rabbit hole" there is a tiny opening of a sebaceous gland which produces sebum, skin's nature-given moisturizer. Pore blockages causing acne form below these openings, deep inside at the epidermis level.

Pores are a natural part of the skin. Fair-skinned models in glossy magazines may look absolutely poreless and flawless. But before you start examining every back dot on your face please remember: a) makeup artists spend hours applying foundations on models' faces starting with primers that visibly reduce the size of pores; b) people with lighter complexions tend to have more narrow pores; 3) there's always such thing as Photoshop. Patch it, blur it, and the pore is gone!

Can we shrink the size of our pores? Unfortunately, no. The size of the pore is hereditary, and nothing really can shrink the pore and alter its physical diameter. Your goal is to keep the pore clean and healthy. When you age, your pore openings will deepen, as skin loses its tautness and elasticity. You can also minimize its appearance with various primers and leave-on treatments.

Sweat

Our body produces two types of fluids that cool, moisturize and cleanse the surface of the skin. If we lived in a perfect world without air pollution, UV radiation and chemically loaded foods, we won't even need all the complex beauty routine—our skin will cleanse, tone and moisturize itself, maybe with a little help of pure water. The perfectly healthy body rarely needs anything else, but let's be realistic. Our skin does require a helping hand from outside.

When everything is working smoothly, the oil ducts send their clear lubricating fluid into the hair follicles that dot your skin (even where you have no hair, you have follicles), and the sweat glands nearby secrete drops of sweat.

Sweat is the most noticeable skin fluid. Every day we sweat out about three cups of sweat off our bodies, no matter how cold or hot there is outside. Sweat is a thin, watery substance. Sweat contains approximately 99% water and 1% solids. The solids are half inorganic salt, mostly sodium chloride, and organic compounds, such as amino acids, urea and peptides.

Sweat helps the body to control temperature but sweat glands are also activated by emotions. That's why we sweat when we are excited or scared! Sweat is also loaded with scented substances that form our unique body odor signature. Human beings are able to communicate on scent level, just like animals, and the odor depends greatly on the physical condition, emotional condition, and of course on sexual desires. There's a suspicion that love on the first sight is actually love on the first sniff!

Sweat also lubricates upper layer skin cells preventing them from shedding too quickly, and here it is getting mixed with oil, or sebum, which is produced by another type of glands, called sebaceous.

Sebum

Sebum is a slightly acidic mixture of oil, water, enzymes and bacteria-fighting blood cells that create a protective film on the skin surface. As a chemical substance sebum is a fat, a triglyceride similar to other organic fats. Most people have the same chemical composition of sebum, and no matter how much sweets you eat you will not alter the formula of your sebum. What you can achieve with sweets or fatty foods is more active production of sebum that flows onto your skin. People with acne usually have more intense sebum production, and the more sebum your skin produces, the worse acne you will experience.

Even though people with problem skin try hard to slow down sebum production and dry it from the skin surface during the day using blotting paper, wipes and towels, sebum is a very useful substance. It's because of sebum our skin can constantly cleanse itself. Due to its slippery oily texture, sebum removes all the debris that otherwise would encrust our skin. Sebum also forms a gentle water-resistant barrier, which is why many water-based lotions for the oily skin don't perform as nicely.

Thanks to sebum, skin is kept naturally moist but can absorb many other ingredients to keep it supple and nourished if they are wrapped in substances friendly to sebum such as oils. That's why nanosome-based serums work better for oily skin.

Sebum also shields our body from attacks of germs, viruses, insects, and fungi that happen 24/7, all year long. Special antiseptic qualities of sebum prevent many skin infections that would occur to us if we dissolve it too vigorously with harsh cleansers and alcohol-based toners.

During certain weather conditions, such as cold or extreme heat, our skin cracks either because the chilled fluids become stiffer and less able to adjust to movement or because they evaporate from skin's surface. In addition to that, low-fat diets also reduce the amount of skin's natural fats, so skin feels dry and chapped. That's why we need moisturizers to maintain the amount of lipids on skin's surface so that skin is able to hold moisture inside.

Unfortunately, sebum is the major contributor to acne. As sebum moves towards the skin surface the triglycerides are split into other substances by the action of the acne-causing bacteria. These substances include fatty acids that can be irritating to the skin. This irritation is important in causing acne.

Sebaceous Glands

Sebaceous glands deliver sebum, an oily mixture of different types of fat, into the follicle, from where it drains to the skin surface.

Depending on the area of your body sebaceous glands can vary in size. The largest sebaceous glands are located at the face, upper back and chest. Those located in the acne-prone areas, such as the face, back and chest, are very large compared to sebaceous glands in other "safe" areas such as legs and hands. Palms of our hand and soles of the feet have no sebaceous glands at all.

Many sebaceous glands have very tiny hairs in them, which not always grow long enough to reach the skin surface. Sebaceous glands, for example, are quite obvious on the nose, even though there is not much hair on it. Sebum tends to block pores with larger, thicker hairs.

The inside wall of the sebaceous gland is covered with epidermal cells which are constantly renewed from the dermis, grow old, flat, and eventually shed when they become completely flat. But they shed inside the pore!

Now sebum comes to rescue. It carries these dead cells away to the skin surface where they are washed or otherwise rubbed off. This is how sebum helps to keep skin clean and healthy. It also keeps the hair follicle moist and supple and hair shiny and smooth. In addition to that, sebum has an acidic nature which helps protect against harmful bacteria.

Sebum starts flowing more actively when we reach puberty. That happens because our bodies begin producing the hormones known as androgens. In terms of acne, the most significant androgen is testosterone, which originates in the testes in men, in the ovaries in women, and in the adrenal glands of both. Through the bloodstream testosterone reaches the hair follicles, where an enzyme manufactured in the skin transforms it into a chemical called dihydrotestosterone—DHT for short. DHT signals the sebaceous glands to start producing sebum.

Can we diminish sebum production with mattifying "oil-absorbing" lotions? Not likely. No matter what you apply to your skin, you cannot change the amount of sebum it produces. No matter how dry or tight they may make your face feel, astringent soaps, lotions, or cosmetics that add more oil on the skin's surface cannot influence sebum output. Nor, contrary to popular belief, do they stimulate the sebaceous gland. Some skincare lines carry oils specifically designed for the oilier skin, for instance, Normalizing Day Oil by German organic skincare label Dr. Hauschka, which is designed "to force" the skin produce less oil because it receives enough oil from outside. Quite simply put, it doesn't work this way.

Only hormones, stress, genetics and diet can regulate the amount of sebum excreted by sebaceous glands, and all cleansers, toners and other topical acne treatments have nothing to do with hormonal balance. What these products can do is to maintain the skin in more or less acceptable state so that sebum doesn't stay inside the pore where it would be dislodged by bacteria.

This is important to understand why using just topical treatments won't help you clearing the acne. Oil production can be affected by diet, stress, genes, and hormones, and it cannot be controlled from outside.

Acne Bacteria

Healthy skin is home to many different kinds of bacteria. These invisible peaceful foreigners protect us from other harmful microorganisms and neutralize some unwanted chemicals. But even these helpful little guys can cause problems if they reproduce too much.

There's one particular type of bacteria that enjoys sebum more than other little creatures. This bacterium is called **_Propionibacterium acnes_**, or P. Acne.

Unlike most bacteria, which eat sugars, these little guys feed on the sebum and produce fatty acids as a waste product. Unfortunately, this waste—call it bacterial poop!—is irritating to the skin. When the body starts producing more sebum, P.

Acne bacteria multiplies in rapid rate, and the more they reproduce, the more bacterial waste they churn out. This "bacterial poop" irritates the skin, body protection mechanism is activated, and we get acne.

However, bacterial discharge is not the only reason we get acne. Skin is a complex and the largest body organ. It's impossible to treat it as if it's separate from other body systems. Skin disorders don't develop due to bacteria or some other external factors. In most cases, many other factors cause acne. To treat it successfully, we must address all these factors, not just visible ones.

LEARN MORE ABOUT ACNE

Everyone can develop acne once in their lifetime. No one is immune to it, unfortunately. Nearly 100% of people suffered from at least an occasional acne outbreak, whether it is a blackhead, whitehead or a full-blown lesion, or zit.

Acne peaks in 85% of young women between the ages of 14 and 16 and in young men between the ages of 16 and 19. Acne affects teenage boys more often than girls because of the production of the male hormone androgen that has a great impact on sebum production. A pimple can suddenly erupt on aging skin of a woman in her menopause. Acne may even hit a newborn in the first few weeks of life when a baby is still under the influence of mother's hormones.

Acne is not a newly invented disease like a seasonal affective disorder. The complete name for acne is *acne vulgaris*, and the origin of the word "acne" dates back more than two thousand years. In ancient Greece the word "acme," which means "point or peak," also meant puberty, which for ancient Greeks with their shorter life span was the peak of life. There is an opinion that actual word "acne" evolved from "acme," as skin blemishes was already a well-known rite of passage for adolescents and young adults.

Today more people get acne than in past decades. According to a survey conducted at University of Leeds (UK), a major center of acne research, the number of women suffering from severe acne increased from 10 percent in 1979 to 14 percent in 1996. Mild acne jumped from 35 percent to 54 percent over the same period, suggesting that more than half of all women today suffer from at least occasional or periodic breakouts.

Acne is so common because everyone has a built-in mechanism for developing it. Acne is natural, and by saying this I don't mean it should be pleasant or funny. Acne happens because our own biochemistry makes it possible.

Acne starts as an inflammation on a cellular level triggered by stress, certain chemicals present in food and skincare products, and hormonal imbalance. For some reason, acne hits hardest when we especially need to feel confident and look good. Acne influences lives of many people, undermining our self-esteem, holding us back from meeting new people, making us fail at job interviews, lose friends and loved ones due to our insecurity and self-doubts.

My own acne history serves as a proof. As a promising TV journalist, I had everything it takes to become a news anchor. With deep insecurity resulting from my ever-present mild to moderate acne and unsightly dark spots, I persuaded everyone including myself that I am not a "camera-friendly" person and that I work much better behind the camera with all the editing, writing, and managing. My low self-esteem along with constant need to upkeep the image of a self-confident professional woman led me to overindulgence in makeup, poor choices in personal life and complete exhaustion by the age of 30. When, by a pure chance, I have discovered the missing link in my skincare approach, the next two years of research has shown that there's something we are all neglecting when taking care of our problem skin.

Even Hollywood stars are suffering from acne. As a matter of fact, they see their dermatologists often and listen to their advice because their incomes depend on their looks. And even if you can retouch and digitally enhance the image on the poster, movie close ups on a big screen tend to reveal all the blemishes and wrinkles. Most stars wear a lot of carefully applied makeup on a daily basis and have a rigorous skin care routine to keep their looking polished and smooth.

Jessica Simpson, Britney Spears, Cameron Diaz and Angelina Jolie all suffer from mild to severe acne and post-acne spots and scars. In one episode of Britney Spears' TV show "Chaotic" she zooms with a home video camera on her acne and comments on her pores. Britney Spears has been featured in ProActive Solutions infomercials in 2005, along with Jessica Simpson. Charlie's Angel Cameron Diaz has been very open about her love of acne-busting Clinique skincare and among her fears she listed being in public without makeup. Angelina Jolie has a beautiful skin but tabloid close-ups reveal "ice pick" acne scars and spots from previous acne that was most likely cleared with her pregnancy.

Bottom line: no one is perfect, we are all humans, and even zillions of dollars and daily facials cannot guarantee you clear skin.

THE MECHANISM OF ACNE

Now that we know the way our skin is built, we can see how acne, skin's most common disorder, actually begins.

Here's a step-by-step process that results in acne:

1. **The pore becomes clogged by dead skin cells**

   As we already know, skin is constantly renewing itself by shedding dead cells off its surface. Sometimes, hormones overstimulate the sebum gland and dead skin cells begin to accumulate inside the pore. Skin cells are rich in protein keratin. When the body produces more sebum, skin start to shed more rapidly, filling the pore.

2. **Dead skin cells mix with large amounts of sebum**

   Our body can produce more sebum than usually due to hormonal tweaks caused by stress, diet or inner changes. The dead skin cells mix with sebum and form a sticky substance that eventually plugs the pore locking its contents inside. A tiny bump called *microcomedo* forms under the skin's surface.

3. **Bacteria multiply inside the pore**

   Very soon, the *Propionibacterium acnes* begin to thrive on this amount of food, and its bacterial discharge makes the inflammation worse. Bacteria consume the sebum and excrete fatty acids. This "bacterial poop" irritates the skin cell walls.

4. **Inflammation increases**

   Acne bacteria contribute to the inflammatory nature of acne by inducing skin cells to secrete proinflammatory cytokines, called *interleukins* and *tumor necrosis factor*. These chemicals can promote inflammation because they attract special "cell killers," or *neutrophils*. This is how pus appears. Blood and lymph swells the nearby areas making them clog and form new comedones which will harbor new portions of acne bacteria. That is why, when we cure one acne pimple, we face a new one, just when we think our job is done.

5. **White substance, or pus, builds on**

   Neutrophils form a primary defense against bacterial infection as they "eat" other cells and foreign substances. The pus in a pimple is made up mostly of neutrophils. In addition, P. acne releases lipases, proteases, and other enzymes which contribute to tissue injury.[12] The inflammation is getting worse. The inflamed pore swells and grows, turns red and inflamed, signaling the birth of a full-size pimple.

   We got used to the idea that pus is bad. In reality, it's the most powerful healing substance that the body can provide. It consists of white blood cells, fibrin, proteins, other infection fighters, fatty cells and water. Don't be tempted to squeeze pus out of the pimple. Squeezing is only helpful when it's time to extract the loosened sebum plug out of the pore which is not swollen and red anymore. We will talk about gentle and effective (and inevitable) squeezing of "ripe" acne pimples later in the book.

6. **Blackhead or whitehead forms**

   If the surface of the pore is too narrow, and air cannot reach the sebum and bacteria broth, then the **whitehead** forms. When the pore is wide enough, the sebum paste containing pigment cells darkens on the air, creating visible black cap, or a **blackhead**. If the blockage of the pore happens only under the skin surface, you see the reddish spot. This is the acne pimple ripening, ready to break out. This spot is tender to touch, and no white cap is visible yet.

7. **Acne is now visible**

   This is when the state of the immune system determines how the acne progresses. If immune response is weak, then the inflammation turns the acne lesion into a whitehead, nodule or even a cyst. Neutrophils will soon clear up the area of inflammation destroying the tissue around the inflamed area.

8. **We panic**

   As soon as we see the red swollen white-tipped bump ripening, we are terrified. The sebaceous gland receives another boost from adrenaline hormone and produces even more sebum, which results in more inflammation. We start applying salicylic acid and benzoyl peroxide, or even topical antibiotics, adding to the irritation and killing white blood cells thus promoting the inflammation. We even try to squeeze the zit, which is especially dangerous at this point. When you squeeze the pimple, you constantly risk to burst the pus in it inwards than outwards, causing the deep inflammation and eventual scarring.

9. **Pimple dries out**

   With or without our help, the area around the pimple will be soon repaired by the body, while the dead neutrophils, dry sebum paste particles and skin cells dry up and eventually shed off, leaving the dark spot from the increased melanin production during the inflammation. However, if the immune system has been weakened, the inflammation can go deeper and pimple evolves into a pustule or a cyst that requires immediate medical attention.

10. **The skin is irritated and weakened by the intense treatment**

   When we apply concentrated doses of benzoyl peroxide, salicylic acid or other traditional acne remedies, skin that already suffers from stress caused by cytokines inside the pimple, becomes weaker. Drying substances in acne treatment lotions encourage surrounding areas of the skin shed faster clogging pores nearby, where they mix with sebum forming new comedones. The vicious circle begins.

HOW DOES ACNE LOOK LIKE?

Those who have acne will instantly recognize it. However, many people mistake acne for perioral dermatitis, rosacea and allergies. There are many spots that only look like acne and really are due to something else. Sometimes acne pimples can take on a quite different appearance.

Let's take a looks at the common attributes of acne. The most important are:

- The increased oiliness of the skin, especially at the T-zone and oilier areas such as upper back and chest;

- The flakiness of the skin and minuscule cracks on the outermost layer of skin (stratum corneum) that are more visible when you apply powder makeup;

- Blackheads that signal the acne formation processes beneath the skin surface;

- Enlarged visible pores, with our without black comedone cap;

- Inflamed blemishes that are red, tender to touch or crowned with white head.

Here are some common characteristics of problem acne-prone skin:

- Your face is shiny (reflects light) in photos

- Your T-zone (nose, chin, forehead) has visible black dots in pores

- Your makeup looks streaky and shiny by midday

- Your skin feels greasy, so you often skip a moisturizer or pick the one that guarantees matte finish

- Your skin always feels comfortable after washing with foaming cleansers and water, even when you use harsh deodorant soap

- You always have red pimples located sporadically at the T-zone, cheeks, jaw line, upper back and chest

- After your acne pimple heals you get a dark spot or even a pitted scar.

TYPES OF ACNE PIMPLES

BLACKHEADS

The formation of blackheads, or comedones, is the earliest stage of acne. Very small blackheads that require a powerful magnifying mirror to be seen are always present even on the healthy skin, while many acne sufferers are "blessed" with easily visible big blackheads located at the t-zone, cheeks and upper back.

Many years ago blackhead tips were thought to be composed of dirt, and acne was supposed to occur in people who didn't wash their faces often enough. However, the black color of blackhead is due to a skin pigment melanin. Pigment producing cells called melanocytes are located at the bottom part of the epidermis and when they are dying and move upwards, they sometimes accumulate in the pore and oxidize becoming black.

Treatment options for blackheads include daily use of AHA (alpha-hydroxy acid) or salicylic acid products, gentle yet thorough cleansing, weekly at-home microdermabrasions and/or at-home glycolic peels. Avoid squeezing the black core because this can lead to redness and scarring. To prevent blackheads from forming whiteheads follow the steps of daily skincare plan suited for your skin type.

WHITEHEADS

Whiteheads form in narrow pores where the content of the pore is blocked inside. Whiteheads look like bumps with white top under the skin. Many people who notice the formation of a whitehead are trying to squeeze it, which then results in increased inflammation and an increased risk of infection and scarring.

Treatment options for whiteheads include topical anti-inflammatory applications along with daily skincare routine for acne-prone skin which will be outlined later in the book. Whiteheads may become the papules if the inflammation progresses.

PAPULES

Papules are red, swollen acne lesions that usually look like small, pink bumps on the skin and can be itchy or tender to the touch. The papules usually last only a few days and when they subside they leave no mark or scar if you resist the temptation to squeeze them out. Some papules may be more visible and harder to the touch. They may persist for some weeks after the noticeable inflammation has gone. Papules may form as a result of contact dermatitis.

Treatment options for papules include topical anti-inflammatory applications along with daily skincare routine for acne-prone skin which will be outlined later in the book. Papules may progress into pustules if the inflammation persists.

PUSTULES

This is the more severe form of papules. Pustules are topped with white head but are more tender to touch and bigger in size than whiteheads. Pustules may also cause throbbing pain in the head or ear depending on their location. The pus may later discharge or in severe cases it has to be incised by the dermatologist and cleared out.

Treatment options for pustules include topical anti-inflammatory applications along with daily skincare routine for acne-prone skin which will be outlined later in the book. If the pain becomes persistent you may try tea tree oil compresses. By all means avoid squeezing the white head out if the pustule is still painful. Pain means that the inflammation is still acute, and by squeezing you will do more harm than good.

NODULES

Nodules, or cysts, are the most critical stage of acne. These are large, painful, pus-filled or solid lesions located deep in the dermis layer with a small opening to the pore. Nodules often feel hard to the touch because they consist of a combination of oils and proteins that have accumulated within the nodular cavity. If left untreated nodules can last for months and leave behind deep crater-like scars.

Treatment options for nodules and acne cysts usually include an aggressive regimen that may include antibiotics. Your dermatologist may recommend injecting corticosteroids into the cyst over a period of 3 to 5 days. Some very large nodular cysts that do not respond to medications may require drainage and surgical excision.

WHAT CAUSES ACNE

Many factors are involved in acne formation. It has been reported that thinner drier skins are more prone to whiteheads and milia because their pores are narrower. Oilier skins almost always have an array of blackheads in the T-zone. Both conditions are in fact inflammatory types of acne that can get worse if triggered by outside factors. Every day we contact thousands and thousands of different chemicals in air, in food, and cosmetics. It's almost impossible to predict when the delicate balance inside the pore is broken and the inflammation begins.

During a study in Croatia, acne was believed to be curable by 96% of acne patients. Most patients (66%) believed that acne would improve immediately after the first treatment; however, the impact of the disease was underestimated by family physicians and also by acne patients. Myths and misconceptions still exist among patients and also among family physicians.[1]

There are many things that can lead to acne flare-ups. Acne is like a time bomb: sometimes all it needs is job interview or a date to flare up and ruin everything. The change of seasons, major moves, such as to another town or even country, wedding, divorce, work stress—all things that set off a wide array of emotions can trigger acne.

Here are the **most common causes of acne**:

Fluctuating Hormone Levels

Hormones play a large part in acne because sebaceous glands are triggered by male hormones androgens, present both in men and women. This is why acne starts to flare up in teenage girls and adult women, most often 5 to 7 days before the menstrual period begins.

The solution: You can balance hormones through diet, clean skincare products, exercise and herbal supplements. We will discuss the ways to normalize hormonal levels later in the book.

Dirt

Dirt does cause acne, even though many acne researchers claim that dirt doesn't cause acne. In fact, 99% of existing acne books and articles declare that neither dirt nor chocolate can contribute to acne. Well, it depends on what we call dirt. By "dirt" we don't mean smudges of mud or greasy patches or streaks of dust on a sweaty face. Dirt consists of airborne particles of soot, smoke, dust, volatile organic compounds, dried sweat, and residue from makeup, sunblocks and skincare. These components pile on the surface of your skin clogging the pores and forming a sticky non-breathable film on top of your skin. As a result, congestion forms deep under the skin surface resulting in acne. **The solution:** You must eliminate the dirt without over-cleansing which may cause skin irritation. We will describe the correct way to double-cleanse your skin using products and techniques designed specifically for each skin type.

Toxic Chemicals

Every day we consume and inhale hundreds of chemical combinations many of which are allergy-causing, hormone-affecting or simply toxic. Some people tend to "break out"—form inflamed red bumps that have mostly allergic nature and don't turn into acne. Sometimes after using a pore-clogging moisturizer or less-than-effective cleanser we develop more visible blackheads that however don't become full-size. However, at a sickly turn of events, a tiny black dot on a cheek may erupt into a volcanic zit overnight just because our skin "didn't like" some mighty doze of chemicals from a sunblock or a mask.

The solution: You have to adopt organic eating habits and avoid eating food loaded with preservatives and other chemical additives if you want to have clear healthy skin. You should also avoid using skincare products containing toxic chemicals whenever possible.

Diet Rich in Saturated Oils and Sugars

Diet rich in sugars and saturated oils cause acne because sugary fatty foods cause fluctuations in sugar levels which in turn stimulates sebaceous glands. Diet rich in shellfish, liver, or spinach that contain high levels of iodine may also stimulate oil production. Dairy is another skin offender because cows are often fed iodine-enriched silage to prevent diseases.

The solution: You have to follow a healthy diet rich in fresh produce and fibers but poor in salts, sugars and refined oils. We will offer you a delicious 30 day Clear Skin Diet later in the book as well as fast exclusive 7-day detox plan to help clear up your skin before an important event.

Yeast Overgrowth

Yeast, a fungus called Candida Albicans, is a normal inhabitant of human digestive tract. Antibiotic use, lack of fiber in the diet, and poor bowel movements may cause yeast to multiply in excess. When yeast overgrows, it emits toxins, most common of which is acetaldehyde, is converted by liver into alcohol and further into sugars. Constant "toxic dump" of Candida causes many health problems, acne among them.

The solution: Maintain a healthy diet low in sugars and processed starches, avoid fermented foods such as vinegars and cured meats that contain yeast, and drink plenty of water. Clear Skin Diet described later in the book helps overcome yeast overgrowth.

Mechanical pressure

Acne can develop from a mechanical irritation or repetitive touching the skin. For example you may develop pimples in the chin area because you may lean your face on the hand, or at the cheek because you press the handset firmly against the cheek, or at the back where you experience rubbing from backpack straps, or at the forehead from the rubbing of the biking helmet.

The solution: You should cleanse your skin thoroughly after the exercise, revise your bad habits and use gauze pads to reduce pressure if you absolutely must wear helmets or other sports equipment.

Certain vitamins and medications

Aspirin, Alka-Seltzer, ibuprofen, Midol, Pepto-Bismol and similar over-the-counter medications as well as vitamin B12 injections, sometimes used to treat anemia, can cause acne. Asthma medications, sedatives, analgesics and cold remedies containing bromides or iodides may contribute to acne flare-ups. Anabolic steroids that are used to grow muscles are a well-known cause of acne in athletes.

The solution: Talk to your doctor about switching to herbal supplements if your medical condition allows it. However, most treatments are temporary so your acne will improve as soon as you stop taking a medication that causes it.

Genes

Acne has a hereditary nature. When both parents have suffered from acne, there are chances three to four that their children will have acne too. The location and severity of acne outbreaks, be it face, chest or upper back, is also genetically inclined. It doesn't mean, however, that if your parents were blessed with clear skin, you are free from acne for life.

The solution: You should adopt new skincare routine as early as possible to avoid permanent damage to your skin.

Picking the Scab

Your skin needs the protective layer of scab to shield the open sore from the outside world. As you will realize later, skin heals from inside out, and when you tear off the healing patch formed by your body over the pimple, it starts forming it again, literally from scratch. Besides, when you pick the scab, you also remove the top layer of newly formed skin cell layer, which results in scarring.

The solution: Never pick the scab, no matter how healed it looks to you. You will never be able to fully disguise the healing pimple under makeup, so at least leave it as it is.

Humidity

Steam baths and saunas should be avoided, because the high temperature and steam cause the blood flow to the affected parts, plus the higher temperature boosts the oil production. You want neither of these things! Unlike the popular belief that steam facial bath opens pores and helps to cure acne, in reality the facial sauna, even with antiseptic additives such as calendula and chamomile, will make the acne turn to worse, even if it seems like it looks better immediately. The cooler and drier you keep your skin, the better for your acne.

The solution: Use blotting papers frequently in the summer to absorb excess oil from the surface of your skin.

Occupation

Occupational acne is most commonly seen in workers exposed to insoluble cutting oils in the machine tool trades or in mechanics exposed to grease and lubricating oils. Some professions aggravate acne due to the person's exposure to certain chemicals. Dielectrics, insecticides, herbicides, fungicides and wood preservatives may cause a very painful form of acne. Exposure to petroleum products and cooking oils may also aggravate acne. Hot humid environments may also cause sufficient hydration and swelling of the skin to predispose to acne. Additional acne-triggering factors include poor hygiene, soiled clothing and lack of adequate washing facilities at the work site.

Women tend to have drier skin and slightly higher skin pH (acidity) than men which may result in higher susceptibility to skin irritants. Women have a greater exposure to irritants within the home on a daily basis such as cleaners, soaps, detergents and waxes which may also contribute to skin irritation. That's why occupational acne occurs more often in women than in men.

The solution: Wash your body quickly after your shift and avoid rubbing your face with dirty hands during the working day. Don't over-wash or you will aggravate acne even more! Powdered soap and waterless cleansers remove greases, tars, paints and some plastics quite easily. Barrier creams also offer a certain amount of protection.

Hairstyling products

Women with long hair sometimes get acne on the neck and upper back. This is caused by the oils from the hair, which may help to clog the pore openings, and possibly by friction of the hair rubbing on the skin. Persistent acne outbreaks along the hairline may appear due to the vigorous brushing with synthetic brush or hair drying with volumizing bristles. Bangs, especially thick ones, can also contribute to acne flare-ups on the forehead. Hairspray, mousses and greasy hair pomades, when constantly applied to the skin at the hairline, can result in clogging the pores and producing new acne lesions.

The solution: Revise your haircare routine and eliminate products one by one until you figure out which one causes you to break out. Then try using products from more natural lines such as Jason, Abba, Aubrey Organics, Prairie Essence, or Giovanni as they all have basic hairstyling products.

IS IT ACNE OR SOMETHING ELSE?

Sometimes we experience a red, itchy rash that looks suspiciously like acne but it flares up in unusual places for acne, such as hands or neck. Even though we are tempted to treat it as acne, in fact these bumps are allergic contact dermatitis, a skin reaction to certain ingredients in jewelry, fragrances or medicine.

Among the "violators" of our skin's health are nickel, which is used in jewelry clasps or buttons, fragrant Balsam of Peru, topical antibiotics, formaldehyde, cobalt chloride found in hair dyes, and Quaternium-15, a preservative often found in hair care products and in industrial paints and polishes. All these chemicals disrupt our health in general, contributing to acne and allergies as well. Dermatitis develops over a longer time and requires a greater amount of an irritant, while allergen causes a reaction almost immediately.

If you suspect that you may have allergic contact dermatitis, you will need to have a skin allergy patch testing to confirm allergies to these substances. You should stay away from anything containing these chemicals—and it is not always possible. For example, formaldehyde contains in most nail polishes, quaternium-15 contains in practically all hair conditioners, and nickel is often used to create white gold in jewellery.

Many women develop skin rashes or bumps when using certain skincare products. Most often, they describe their reaction as "It breaks me out" or "It burns my face." This happens when you develop a minor allergic reaction to one or more ingredients in this product. Something in the formulation simply throws your skin off balance. It might happen not because the formula is bad—due to your unique biochemistry you may simply not tolerate some ingredients or their combinations. Skin can also develop acne-like bumps because certain ingredients tend to concentrate in the pores when applied to skin (ever noticed moisturizer soaking into pores?) and because of higher concentration of the product in the pore fragile thin walls inside get irritated faster, resulting in a red pimple.

If you start treating your dermatitis "breakouts" as if it was acne, you will only worsen things. Instead, try to be as gentle as possible. Revise your skincare routine and exclude the new product that you just purchased, at least for a few days. Apply compress made of gauze soaked in cool chamomile or green tea, allow it to dry and remove the gauze. You may apply a cream containing hydrocortisone to relieve redness and itching. Avoid scratching or picking the bump at all means!

WHY ZIT ZAPPERS FAIL

It takes 14 days for the acne pimple to form underneath the skin surface, while the complete turnaround of the skin takes 28 to 35 days. This means that during this period we may still have nasty pimples that still hide beneath, even after we have cleared the surface. Now you see why all those 3-day acne-free schemes are a phony!

For the same reason topical blemish spot treatments only conceal the problem, doing nothing to fighting the acne itself. Benzoyl peroxide, tea tree oil, and other antiseptic concoctions used alone sometimes create only more irritation and swelling.

The acne blemish forms underneath the skin surface for several weeks, and trying to zap it on the surface is the same as trying to melt the tip of the iceberg—the real problem lies deep under water.

No matter what kind of zit "zapper" you tried in the past, be it clay masks, toothpaste, tea tree oil, patches, or topical antibiotics, I am sure you didn't prevent the future breakouts from forming underneath your skin. Even worse, many of these pimple spot treatments contain irritating ingredients that damage the skin, which only worsens the natural healing process of acne. Many, if not most, spot treatments contain drying and sensitizing components, which lead to dehydration and premature aging of your skin.

As simple as the formation of acne sounds, it doesn't mean that killing the bacteria and clearing up the pore will improve your condition. More often, though, acne remains and flare-ups keep on … well, flaring up.

This is because the very functioning of your body systems causes acne to flare. When your immune system is weak, acne bacteria cause more damage because the healing of the pimple is extremely slow. The right acne treatment should start with detoxifying your body, calming your nerves, balancing hormones and strengthening the immune system.

If you continue dealing only with surface outbreak of the acne ignoring the complex process that lies underneath, you will never prevent acne pimples or post-acne scarring. Following all the steps of your daily skincare routine you will deal not only with the tip of the iceberg, but with all the stages of acne blemish formation, which will allow you to stop further breakouts and prevent them from occurring.

Luckily for us, setting your body working in the right direction is easier than you think. It takes a little, really. Everyone can do it, and if you are reading this far, you are smart enough to clear your skin and stop those nasty blemishes from ruining your life!

ACNE IS NOT CONTAGIOUS

Acne is not an "infection" in the true sense of the word. Acne and blemishes are not a contagious disease, transmitted by microbes, that one person can catch from another. The bacteria that are involved are normal inhabitants of the skin that become troublesome only when favorable conditions permit them to multiply excessively in the follicles. So you don't need to fear that you will develop acne if you touch, share food with, or kiss someone who has it.

Although we don't know all the details of the way the bacteria are involved in acne we are pretty certain about one point. That is, they are not infecting the skin in the same way that other bacteria do, for example, when they cause a boil, impetigo or an infected cut. You can't catch acne—if you could, all dermatologists (skin specialists) would have it all the time!

Some researchers claim that acne blemishes aren't all bad news. Doctors suggest that sufferers of acne may be protected to some degree against skin cancer by the very same bacteria which causes acne. "One day we may all be popping pills of P.acne in a bid to stay healthy!" said Dr Anne Eady at University of Leeds' skin research unit.

WHY YOU MUST TREAT YOUR ACNE

Acne is a skin condition that affects more than our looks. In most cases, acne is a result of hormonal disturbance, stress, metabolism disorder, or other factors. You should understand that acne has many underlying causes, and there are many treatments available should your acne be caused by hormonal imbalance, stress or poor diet. In the next chapters you will learn how to treat your acne by eliminating stress, by balancing your hormones, by adjusting your diet and lifestyle. Most importantly, you will learn how to care for your acne-prone skin at any age, in any situation.

According to the new research, only 30 percent of acne sufferers seek medical treatment. Not many adults who have jobs, families and many chores to do on a daily basis have time to attend their pimples. Most women prefer to slap on some concealer on their pimples, instead of trying to get rid of them. People with acne are often emotionally challenged, and numerous studies reveal that acne sufferers are prone to neuroticism, psychosomatic condition, social extraversion, and self-defensive attitude, as well as the social anxiety[2].

Once you've met yourself, inside and out, you've got no excuse for using the wrong medicine or the wrong approach. As you go through the thirty-day program you must pay constant attention to changes in your skin. As your skin clears up, it will gain new sensitivities. As you use stronger and stronger acne treatments, watch for over-drying and excessive redness. Be flexible in your approach. You may need to change remedies, to experiment with techniques. The regimen in this book is designed for you to use by yourself at home. So take charge of your skin. You've got everything to gain!

TRADITIONAL OPTIONS FOR ACNE

Skin is in constant contact with the outside world, and it needs extra care to stay beautiful and healthy. Unfortunately, many conventional treatments for clear acne-free skin actually work against skin's health, disrupting its abilities to repair and protect itself. In fact, many traditional acne treatments increase acne by flaring up the inflammation in the pimple and in a surrounding skin, making it more sensitive and prone to various infections and attacks from outside world.

Prescription and over-the-counter acne medications contain various concentrations of basic anti-acne ingredients such as benzoyl peroxide, vitamin A acids, salicylic acid, glycolic acid and rarely sulfur. Let's take a look at conventional acne treatments and their positive and negative aspects.

WHAT'S WRONG WITH BENZOYL PEROXIDE?

Benzoyl peroxide (BP) is the main ingredient in the vast majority of chemical-based acne treatments available over the counter, and some sources claim that this chemical can treat 100 per cent of all acne cases. As an acne treatment, benzoyl peroxide has been widely used since 1930s. There are many cleansing liquids, bars, lotions, and creams with several strengths of benzoyl peroxide available on the market, from 2.5 per cent in over-the-counter drugs and up to 10 per cent in acne medications available by prescription only.

Benzoyl peroxide works against acne in a multitude of ways. As an antiseptic, it kills P.Acne bacteria working in a different way than antibiotics. As an oxidizing agent and an anti-inflammatory benzoyl peroxide helps to dry out acne pimples on the skin surface. Many companies market complete skincare kits based on benzoyl peroxide containing cleansers, treatment astringents and topical creams with different percentage of BP.

Benzoyl peroxide has long been known to be an allergen and a strong irritant. It may cause skin's dryness and increase skin's sensitivity, but it's usually better tolerated by people with oilier, thicker skin. Benzoyl peroxide, like most peroxides, is a powerful bleaching agent, and may cause uneven pigmentation in people with darker skin. Since benzoyl peroxide removes the top layer of the skin, it also increases sun sensitivity and premature aging, so a strong SPF is recommended if you decide to go for this kind of treatment. In some cases, benzoyl peroxide can cause severe facial swelling and itchiness that go away when the benzoyl peroxide treatment is discontinued[3].

Due to its oxidizing action, benzoyl peroxide is a potent free radical-generating compound. Free radical generating compounds have been shown to speed up the malignant conversion of papillomas to carcinomas in skin.

In many studies, benzoyl peroxide promoted both papillomas and carcinomas[4]. In animal studies, benzoyl peroxide has been shown to promote carcinomas, or skin tumors[5, 6], and promote other types of cancer such as lymph nodes cancer, in another study[7]. In studies, animals were treated with up to 20% benzoyl peroxide preparation for up to 5 months.

While people with acne don't always use concentrated benzoyl peroxide, they tend to stick to their blemish zappers for years, and no one has ever studied the cumulative effect which may result from a prolonged exposure to benzoyl peroxide even in smaller doses. However, benzoyl peroxide is recommended for consistent use on a long term basis.

In the U.S., FDA indicated that benzoyl peroxide was safe to use until 1995. Later, FDA has revised its decision and classified benzoyl peroxide as "safety uncertain."[8] The federal agency is now insisting that all products containing benzoyl peroxide should carry safety warnings. Despite many years of use, benzoyl peroxide has also never been tested on pregnant women. Needless to say, it's not recommended to use during pregnancy.

Since 2003, benzoyl peroxide, along with hydroquinone, has been banned for use in cosmetics sold in the European Union. Benzoyl peroxide preparations may be bought at the pharmacy or the chemist, most often by prescription only[9].

Of course, not all people who diligently use benzoyl peroxide for years will develop skin cancer. However, would you want to use a product which safety is unknown for several years only to learn about the harm that you were causing to your body all this time?

SALICYLIC ACID

Salicylic acid is your best ally when fighting acne, especially if you are past teen-age years. Also known as Beta Hydroxy Acid, salicylic acid is the key ingredient in many skin-care products such as cleansers, lotions, and toners, all available over the counter.

The very action of salicylic acid is unique. It dissolves skin cells, and that's why salicylic acid is so beneficial for treating acne: due to its little molecular weight it penetrates deeply into a pore dissolving the build-up of dead skin cells, stubborn sebum and hair particles. This allows the sebum flow in a healthy way, draining freely onto a skin surface. Finally, salicylic acid which is chemically related to aspirin, is an anti-inflammation agent that can help calm down the red-ness of pimples.

Working as a dead cell remover, salicylic acid when used in form of a wash or a lotion eases the penetration of other useful anti-acne ingredients, such as tea tree oil and other substances. Salicylic acid is also a powerful antiseptic with anti-oxidant and anti-inflammatory properties. When you use it daily, it will not only open pore clogging, but will also reduce swelling and dissolve those little come-dones that started forming.

Salicylic acid can be used in relatively high concentrations, although when used in excess, it can dry skin and make it too sensitive. Some people are allergic to salicylic acid, and they should stop using it immediately.

As of the moment of writing, I have not found any studies of salicylic acid in pregnant women, however there were no problems reported on salicylic acid use on nursing babies in case of acne in newborns. High doses of the acid in its oral form have been shown in studies to cause birth defects and various pregnancy complications. Make sure your doctor knows if you are pregnant or if you may become pregnant, especially if you will be using salicylic acid in high concentra-tions or to treat body acne. Always discuss the risks and benefits of any acne treat-ment with your doctor.

Because salicylic acid is not water-soluble, many of the products containing it are formulated with high concentrations of alcohol, which can irritate acne-prone skin. Also remember that salicylic acid is effective only at concentrations of at least 1%, preferably 2%, and in an acid base, with a pH (acidity) level between 3 and 4.

SULFUR

Sulfur is the oldest acne medication used since 1800s. It is a powerful drying and peeling agent that works by reducing bacteria and helping unclog pores. Today, sulfur is not the most popular skincare ingredient due to its unpleasant odor. Sulfur is most often used in soaps, such as Stiefel Sulfur Soap, and other facial cleansers, or masks, such as Sulfur Therapeutic Mask with Aloe Vera and sulfur by DDF. Blemish Clearing Serum by Juice Beauty is a truly natural gem with amazing organic ingredients and quite potent sulfur.

PRESCRIPTION SOLUTIONS

If you have severe acne that resists non-prescription treatments, you may want to see a dermatologist. Prescription antibiotic topical and oral treatments and retinoid preparations are the acne treatments of choice for many, and doctors usually prescribe oral antibiotics only if more gentle methods fail to resolve the problem.

Please note that systemic acne treatments harm the whole body while only temporarily clearing the skin, so make sure to explore more gentle ways of clearing acne before you try antibiotics or retinoids. Acne medications must be taken for several months before you notice the improvement in your acne condition.

Topical Retinoids

Retinoids treat acne by increasing cell turnover which helps unplug blocked pores. Vitamin A acid preparations, or Retin-A, have been used to treat acne since 1960s. Retinoids work by increasing skin cell turnover promoting the release of the plugged material in the pore thus preventing the formation of new comedones. Retinoids may be quite irritating and can even increase the inflammation in the acne lesion. The acne can worsen during the first month of treatment because the medication draws out the eruptions hiding in deeper layers of the skin. Another downside is that retinoid preparations can dry out the skin making it sensitive to outside aggressions and bacteria. Because they work by thinning the skin, retinoids also increase risk of sunburn.

With retinoids, results can sometimes begin in as little as one week, but most often takes 4 to 6 weeks to really notice improvement.

Retinoids are available as liquids (most potent form), gels, and creams (less potent form). The best-known topical retinoid is known as Retin-A, Avita, and Renova. A new formulation Retin-A Micro 0.1% releases retinoid over a longer period of time and is less irritating. Retin-A must be used at night because it's deactivated by the sun.

Newer topical retinoid Adapalene (Differin) causes less skin irritation than tretinoin and is stable in the presence of benzoyl peroxide. Tazarotene (Tazorac) works the same way and just as effectively, but is more expensive. Both these medications can be used any time of the day.

Advantage: topical retinoids provide the relief from acne as well as help fading of acne marks and other skin discolorations.

Disadvantages: a lot of mild to moderate side effects which most commonly include stinging, burning, redness, peeling, scaling, or discoloration and dryness of the skin leading to premature aging. Patients should report prolonged or severe side effects to their doctor. The skin starts to improve after 4 to 8 weeks, and acne often reoccurs after the treatment is discontinued.

Accutane

Oral retinoid Accutane (isotretinoin) is usually reserved for severe acne, especially on the back and chest. Doctors prescribe it when all other solutions have been tried without much success. Oral retinoids reduce sebum production as well as excessive production of skin cells in the lining of the pore. During oral isotretinoin therapy, sebum production is reduced by 90% or more. Retinoids do not have any antibacterial properties but because they greatly reduce the amount of serum produced by the skin bacteria doesn't multiply. According to a study, more than 38% of Accutane patients remained acne-free for three years or more.

Advantage: Accutane does provide long-term relief for severe nodular or cystic acne.

Disadvantages: side effects can be quite severe. First of all, retinoids are known to cause severe birth defects, so any treatment must be completed at least three months before you plan to get pregnant. At least two ways of contraception must be used when on Accutane. Other side effects are just as bad: Accutane may cause inability to see in the dark, intracranial pressure, and liver problems. Regular blood tests must be performed regularly to check on liver function. Retinoids when taken by mouth can produce severe dryness, itching and peeling of the facial skin. Dryness around the mouth, lips, nose, in the eyes and on eyelids is also quite common. Nosebleeds are also quite common and the application of petroleum jelly is recommended. Retinoids may cause depression but this link has not been proven, as severe acne itself can cause anxiety and depression. However, there has been a joint effort on the part of families whose children have committed suicide while on Accutane to try to get this medication off the market.

Accutane treatment can last for up to 16 weeks and if there is a relapse, a second course of treatment may be prescribed by your dermatologist. Retinoid therapy is expensive and is available only via the supervision of a dermatologist. Consult with your physician and be advised by his or her recommendations.

Antibiotics

Topical antibiotics are a starting point of prescription acne therapy. Antibiotics help stop or slow the growth of bacteria and reduce inflammation and swelling.

Antibiotics can be prescribed in oral or topical form. The two main topical antibiotics used in acne are erythromycin and clindamycin in form of gels, creams, lotions, and wipes. Antibiotics for topical use can be formulated alone or in combination with benzoyl peroxide or zinc.

Oral antibiotics are used to treat moderate to severe inflammatory acne over the past 40 years. Oral antibiotics work by reducing the number of P. acnes and Staphylococcus in the skin. Oral antibiotics are usually prescribed for at least 6 to 8 weeks with a maximum of four to six months. Antibiotic treatment requires consistency. You should never interrupt treatment and take the prescribed dose regularly or the treatment becomes ineffective. Make sure to review with your doctor all the medications you are taking including over-the-counter and herbal supplements to avoid problems with drug interactions.

Advantages: oral antibiotics provide long-time relief from acne that is not responsive to topical treatments.

Disadvantages: side effects for topical antibiotics include stinging, burning, dryness, contact dermatitis, peeling, itching, and redness. The most common side effects of oral antibiotics include upset stomach and nausea. Some antibiotics are more prone to cause some of the side effects than others. Pseudo-membranous colitis is a potentially serious intestinal problem that can uncommonly be caused by clindamycin. Tetracycline is not given to pregnant women, nor is it given to children under 8 years of age because it might discolor developing teeth. Tetracycline and minocycline may also decrease the effectiveness of birth control pills.

A new study shows that people treated with antibiotics for acne for more than six weeks were more than twice as likely to develop an upper respiratory tract infection within one year as individuals with acne who were not treated with antibiotics. Within the first year of observation, 15 percent of the patients with acne had at least one common infectious illness, upper respiratory tract infection, and within that year, the odds of having this infection among those receiving antibiotic treatment were 2.15 times greater than among those who were not receiving antibiotic treatment, the study by David J. Margolis, M.D., Ph.D., of the University of Pennsylvania School of Medicine, Philadelphia, shows.

Other studies have compared the efficacy and cost effectiveness of different treatment options for acne—including the comparison of tablet antibiotics and antibiotic lotions with the antimicrobial treatment benzoyl peroxide.

"Differences in cost-effectiveness between regimens were large; the cheapest treatment (benzoyl peroxide) was 12 times more cost-effective than minocycline. We found that clinical efficacy of oral tetracyclines is compromised by pre-existing propionibacterial resistance. By contrast, topical regimens that included erythromycin and benzoyl peroxide were unaffected by resistance but were not superior to benzoyl peroxide alone," says professor Hywel Williams from the Universities of Nottingham and Leeds, UK.

Oral Contraceptives

Acne typically first appears during adolescence and can persist well into adulthood. The cause of acne is most often linked to androgens, which are the hormones that stimulate the sebaceous—or oil—glands in the skin. When the sebaceous glands are over-stimulated by androgens, acne flare-ups can occur.

For women affected by acne, especially those in the early-to-mid twenties and older, oral contraceptives (OCPs) can be an effective part of their acne treatment plan in conjunction with other therapies. Current oral contraceptives help decrease androgen levels, and therefore decrease acne.

Oral contraceptives seem to work best in women with oilier skin whose acne flares before their menstrual periods and consists of painful, often deep, inflammatory acne lesions. Oral contraceptives are a combination of synthetic estrogen and progestin, two female sex hormones. Combinations of estrogen and progestin work by preventing ovulation (the release of eggs from the ovaries). They also change the lining of the uterus to prevent pregnancy from developing and change the mucus at the cervix to prevent sperm from entering.

However, increased sebum production is only one cause of acne, and doctors may also prescribe oral medications or topical creams, gels, or lotions with vitamin A derivatives, benzoyl peroxide, or antibiotics to help unblock the pores and reduce bacteria. All together, this course of treatment has an incredible load on woman's body, especially kidneys and liver.

Advantages: most women whose acne has hormonal nature see the improvement over the first three months. Birth control pills are also effective for other medical conditions such as endometriosis, polycystic ovarian syndrome (PCOS) and fibrocystic breast conditions. Many women experience fewer symptoms of PMS while using oral contraceptives.

Disadvantages: the most serious side effect of oral contraceptive pills is tromboembolism (blood clots), most commonly the deeper veins in the legs. Other side effects include dizziness, headache, lightheadedness, stomach upset, bloating, nausea and weight gain.[20] There may be an increased risk of breast cancer and cervical cancer in women who use oral contraceptives for more than five years.

Laser and Light Therapies

New laser and light treatments can specifically target two of the factors that cause acne. While lasers can thermally reduce the oil production of the sebaceous glands and light sources can destroy acne bacteria itself, lasers designed to target only inflammatory acne and are not effective for people who have only black-heads or whiteheads. Photodynamic therapy, a light-based treatment, uses the combination of a photosensitizing medication on the skin that is then treated with a light to target the oil glands and P. acnes bacteria. Both of these therapies reduce the overproduction of oil which helps diminish and in some cases completely remove acne.

Resurfacing with a laser is considered ablative (such as CO2) which is more intense, and non-ablative (NLite) which involves heat-induced fibroblast stimulation to thicken the underlying collagen structure.

Non-ablative laser treatments are commonly used to treat acne and post-acne scars and marks. One of the main benefits of non-ablative lasers, in contrast to their ablative counterparts, is that they deliver the amount of infrared energy to trigger a thermal wound response but without the harmful effects to the epidermis.

Non-ablative laser resurfacing is performed by dermatologists and plastic surgeons during a series of treatments. The yellow light of non-ablative laser passes right through the epidermis generating heat in and around the sebaceous glands and creating a mild thermal injury. This stimulates your own dermis to produce its own natural collagen. By just below the skin's surface, a non-ablative laser alters the structure and function of the sebaceous gland, leading to prolonged acne clearance. There is no downtime and no side effects except for mild bruising and swelling.

The 532-nm potassium titanyl phosphate laser, 585- and 595-nm pulsed dye lasers, 1450-nm diode laser, and 1540-nm erbium glass laser have been used to treat acne, often in combination with other therapies. Potential drawbacks associated with lasers include potential pain, skin discoloration, and cost of treatment[12]. Lasers can decrease pigmentation in darker skin tones so the treatment may not be suitable for people with these skin types. There are only a few laser devices, such as ClearLight, the Aura laser and Aurora which combines intense pulsed light with radiofrequency, were found suitable for treating acne in dark skin tones.

Intense pulsed light and blue light are used during **photodynamic acne therapy**. During the treatment, the device creates a series of bright light flashes of various spectrum color which kills acne bacteria in case of blue light, and improve skin texture, tone, pore size and collateral collagen building in case of intense pulsed light. In addition to that, photodynamic therapy using a topical medication called aminolevulinic acid (Levulan) has been approved by FDA to treat actinic keratosis, an early potential sign of skin cancer.[13]

Advantages: there are no severe side effects associated with lasers compared to systemic acne therapies. Laser treatments help achieve clear and more youthful skin that will look perfectly natural. Non-ablative laser therapy is also being used to successfully treat the scars that remain long after the initial acne has been cleared. There is no downtime and no preparation required.

Disadvantages: non-ablative lasers may cause swelling and redness of the areas treated. Following the treatment by laser or intense pulsed light, your skin will be red and sensitive, and redness will probably persist for several weeks. During the treatment you should avoid sun and use sunblocks with highest SPF available. The whole course of laser treatment is quite costly (from $1200 to $4000 depending on the area treated and the type of laser used) and may not be covered by your insurance. Your specialist may also recommend further therapy six to 12 months after your first treatment.

It may seem that laser and light treatments for acne can make other acne treatments unnecessary which would certainly benefit all concerned—except cosmetics companies. But doctors are not yet at the point where acne patients are going to throw out their medicated lotions and line up for the laser. Most studies on laser therapy for acne have been small and not meticulously designed. But because the laser treatment devices don't generally cause harm to patients, many dermatologists are using lasers in clinical practice based on these early studies.

Chemical Peels

Chemical peels are becoming a popular treatment for acne and scarring. During chemical peel the pores are cleared from blockages as the acid in the peel causes top layer of the skin to scrap off. After the peel the regeneration process in the skin speeds up which causes pores to shrink and scars fade. There are several different solutions available for chemical peels, and they each have their advantages and disadvantages. There are several solutions used in chemical peels: glycolic acid, salicylic acid, Jessner's solution and trichloroacetic acid.

Glycolic acid is used for light chemical peels that do not penetrate beyond the upper layers of the skin. Light peels help correct surface scarring and diminish acne. **Salicylic acid** is chemically related to Aspirin and is commonly used in concentrations from 20% to 30%. It penetrates the skin pores more easily and has an anti-inflammatory effect which makes it ideal peel for acne. There is also usually more noticeable skin smoothing and decrease in inflammation after a salicylic acid treatment than with glycolic acid.[14]

Trichloroacetic acid is the oldest light peel and it is considered safe and helpful in case of acne spots and marks. It can be used in strengths from 5% approximately 20% to achieve a superficial peel. Trichloroacetic acid peels in concentrations above 50% allows for more active peeling but can result in scarring, so this treatment should be made only in a dermatologist office. For this reason, be cautious about TCA peel kits available over the Internet.

Jessner's peel is a medium peel containing 14% salicylic acid, 14% lactic acid, and 14% resorcinol. There's a serious controversy over the safety of this solution as resorcinol has been reported in European studies as a potent allergen[26] and lactic and salicylic acid act as penetration enhancers allowing for better absorption of resorcinol by the body.

Between the peels you should carefully avoid the sun and use sunblocks with high SPF (recommended creams: La Roche-Posay Anthelios 60 XL Cream, Dr. Hauschka Sunscreen Cream for Children SPF 22). After the treatment you may wish to apply a healing barrier cream to soothe and protect the skin (recommended products: Weleda Skin Food, Jurlique Herbal Recovery Mist AG.)

Advantages: chemical peels provide surface relief from acne but they do a great job in fading acne marks and evening out acne scars. In addition to that, chemical peels diminish other skin discolorations and help firm the aging skin and smooth out wrinkles.[28] Peelings can be done on all skin types, and there is no downtime and no preparation required.

Disadvantages: peeling compounds can cause swelling and stinging when applied. Light peels should be performed in a course over four to six weeks and a maintenance program to keep acne under control is required.

Microdermabrasion

Microdermabrasion is basically an intense scrub. The device blasts a controlled flow of aluminum oxide crystals that scrub off the very top layer of the skin and are sucked away by the same tube. Microdermabrasion works well for acne marks and skin discolorations but for pitted acne scars you would need to undergo a **dermabrasion**, a deeper treatment that penetrates epidermis layer of the skin. While microdermabrasion is available at spa and beauty salons, deep dermabrasion should only be performed by a dermatologist.

There are many **at-home microdermabrasion** kits available today such as L'Oreal Dermo-Expertise ReFinish Micro-Dermabrasion Kit, Neutrogena Advanced Solutions At-Home MicroDermabrasion System and Estee Lauder Idealist Micro-D Thermal Refinisher. Most of them contain aluminum oxide crystals in a cream that should be rubbed manually or using an electric rotating device. To minimize your exposure to chemicals we recommend derma e Microdermabrasion Scrub that delivers buffing aluminum oxides in organic blend of essential oils and vitamin E.

Advantages: microdermabrasion is a "lunchtime" moderately priced procedure as there is no downtime and the redness and irritation are minimal. The skin looks more taut and smooth, pores are temporary cleared and acne marks and spots are faded after four to six procedures. When the top dead skin cell layer is exfoliated, topical treatments can penetrate better.

Disadvantages: results are not long-lasting. While acne spots and marks may fade forever, pores will become clogged in the matter of weeks. Maintenance treatments are required every six to eight weeks for best results. Dermabrasion results in more radical chances but may sometimes cause skin discolorations, swelling, inflammation and even scarring.

Cryotherapy

Cryotherapy is another form of peel that uses freezing liquids such as liquid nitrogen or solid carbon dioxide to reduce skin temperature to very low levels. This low temperature causes the top layer of skin to shed, eliminating acne and reducing inflammation. These procedures are becoming less popular as newer treatments become available.

Advantages: there is no medication and no chemicals involved, and in many cases acne is greatly diminished within weeks of regular treatments.

Disadvantages: side effects of cryotherapy include stinging and redness of the skin. In rare instances, the skin may swell and blister after a cryotherapy treatment.

After a review of most common prescription acne drugs and dermatologist-performed procedures it's easy to see that most of them carry a lot of risks and pose a lot of serious side effects. Only non-ablative laser treatments offer additional benefits such as decrease in skin's aging. However, doctors reveal that even when prescribing these drugs, they still wander in the dark about why acne actually happens and what to do when it starts.

In the past, intensive procedures targeted only the pimples themselves while causing premature aging by drying out and sensitizing the skin. Today, the new concept of acne treatment suggests that the entire body should be treated. Even if your skin appears normal on the surface, the acne may be developing underneath. This means that your skin should be treated as part of your body in order to avoid the acne from occurring in the first place.

Changes in sleep cycles, diet, relationships, and events in our lives—both good and bad—all affect our physical health. Our bodies are constantly adapting both internally and externally to changes within our bodies and in the world around us. Chemical peels, microdermabrasion and other targeted procedures only help repair past damage. They are not the solution to your acne problem. If you want to have clear skin, your main goal is to prevent the acne blemish from forming. You can achieve it by following the Clear Skin Diet, practicing stress-reducing fitness routine and using clean skincare products that contain no harmful toxic ingredients that disrupt the health of your skin.

CLEAR SKIN FROM INSIDE

Your unique skin structure, your lifestyle and eating habits, your emotional state and preferences in skincare and makeup all contribute to acne. No matter when acne strikes you in your teenage years or in your 40s, there is a solution, and it's sweeter than you thought.

First of all, we invite you to revise your eating habits. It has been proven that food does contribute to acne, and food can also help cure it. In the next chapter we will explain why eating habits can ruin or save your skin. We will introduce you to the Clear Skin Diet and a crash-course Clear Skin Detox plan that helps you improve your skin condition in days before an important event. This three-day detox is an intense fad diet and it should be only used in emergency situations!

Secondly, we will explain how stress contributes to your acne. We will suggest you a simple plan to decrease your stress levels without resorting to prescription medications. This plan will help you invigorate your skin and calm down your nerves so that you sleep better and wake up with glowing complexion.

Thirdly, we will go into your skincare routine. You will learn which chemical ingredients in your skincare and makeup contribute to your acne by disrupting your endocrinal and immune balance and which ingredients can actually harm your health increasing your chances for getting cancer and other fatal illnesses. We will suggest a number of cleansers, toners, moisturizers and topical treatments suitable for your specific skin condition and we will also share some exclusive simple recipes for homemade acne treatments that will literally cost you pennies!

Every day we receive emails from happy readers of the previous e-book edition of Clear Acne Guidebook who share their stories of success and even offer their own tips and solutions to ongoing skin woes. You too can soon get rid of acne for life and enjoy healthy glowing—and younger—skin.

CLEAR SKIN WITH HERBS AND VITAMINS

In treating acne, many herbs and vitamins work by boosting immune and elimination body systems while gently regulating hormonal levels. Immune system is responsible for protection from diseases. When this immune system weakens, our body starts showing symptoms of various disorders, such as acne. There are many factors that affect our immune system, but some major factors include antibiotic overuse and misuse, pollution, environmental toxins, stress, emotional disturbance, and lifestyle.

Vitamin A

Vitamin A aids in hormone production, maintains the integrity of mucous membranes and the digestive tract, and is beneficial for night vision. Vitamin A also helps in the growth of skin, teeth, bone and improves immune system function. In addition to that, vitamin A is a powerful antioxidant responsible for the health of cell membrane and protection of it from harmful radicals. Vitamin A belongs to a group of carotenoids which can be found in its natural state in eggs, orange, red and green leafy vegetables such as red bell peppers, spinach, watercress broccoli, cantaloupe, carrots, and also in cod and halibut.

In some cases, very large doses of vitamin A have been successfully used to treat severe acne[15]. The recent study shows that intake of vitamin A and E by people suffering from acne was shown to improve their acne condition[16]. In addition, doctors found that there is a strong relationship between decrease in vitamin A levels in the body and increase in the severity of acne condition. But you must remember that higher doses of vitamin A which is related to isotretinoin (Accutane) can be very toxic to the body and it should be taken only under supervision of a doctor. It happens because this vitamin is fat soluble and if taken in large amounts it gets stored in the body, unlike water soluble vitamins which are excreted easily. Do not take additional vitamin A supplement if you are pregnant.

Vitamins of B group

The vitamins in the B complex are thiamine, riboflavin, niacin (nicotinic Acid, niacinamide), pantothenic acid, pyridoxine and cyanocobalamin. Each one of these vitamins has a specific role in promoting healthy skin, as well as overall health. Thiamine (vitamin B1) acts as an antioxidant while enhancing circulation and assisting in proper digestion. Riboflavin (Vitamin B2) works together with vitamin A to maintain and improve the mucous membranes in the digestive tract.

It is also essential for healthy skin, hair and nails. Acne is a symptom of riboflavin deficiency.

Niacinamide (vitamin B3) is vital for healthy skin. It works by improving circulation and helping your body with the metabolism of carbohydrates, fats and proteins. Also known as niacin, vitamin B3 helps the body synthesize healthy amounts of hormones by regulating hormone levels, particularly during menstrual cycles and menopause.

Vitamin B6 is perhaps the most powerful anti-acne vitamin in B-group. Because of its metabolic properties and hormonal supporting role, vitamin B6 (pyridoxine) is great for the immune system. A deficiency of vitamin B6 can result in acne. During a research involving adolescent girls who had menstruation difficulties, vitamin B6 intake has reduced symptoms of acne by 50-75%. However, the excessive intake of vitamin B can aggravate acne. Another study reports that inflamed lesions resembling acne rosacea were temporally associated with daily ingestion of high-dose B vitamin supplement[17]. Everything is good in moderation.

Vitamin E

Vitamin E is a powerful antioxidant that promotes healing and tissue repair. Through its antioxidant and anti-inflammatory effects, topical vitamin E may enhance wound healing, although the benefits remain controversial[18]. Vitamin E also helps protect red blood cells and is important for the proper function of nerves and muscles. If you suffer from PMS, this vitamin will reduce breast tenderness, nervous tension, headache, fatigue, depression, and insomnia as symptoms of PMS. Vitamin E works against acne in close connection with vitamin A. A study shows that by adding vitamin E to the diet the vitamin A doctors controlled acne with more success, even where vitamin A alone had failed[19].

Zinc

Zinc is perhaps the most famous acne fighter among minerals. Zinc is an essential trace element for the human organism that reduces inflammation, helps immune function, and keeps hormone levels in check. Zinc functions in more enzymatic reactions than any other mineral! Zinc woks by increasing the level of white blood cells which are important in fighting off infections caused by bacteria. That's why zinc has proved to be very beneficial in treating acne. Studies have shown that in case of acne, zinc shows the same results as erythromycin. During the newest study in Europe, thirty patients with inflammatory acne were treated by zinc gluconate with a daily dose of 30 mg for two months. In vivo, this study displayed a reduction in the number of inflammatory lesions after a 2-month treatment whether or not acne bacteria was active[20]. During different studies doses varied from 30 to 150 mg of elemental zinc, but all studies have shown that might be an alternative treatment when antibiotics are not recommended[21].

The toxicity of zinc is very low, except for when it is taken at high doses (more than 200 mg of zinc gluconate or 30 mg of elemental zinc) for a long period of time. Zinc is not teratogenic and can be given during pregnancy. Major side effects are abdominal with nausea and vomiting. Zinc is found naturally in generous amounts in brewers yeast, whole grains, Brazil nuts and pumpkin seeds. All these ingredients can easily become part of your daily diet with our Clear Skin Diet which is outlined later in the book.

Essential Fatty Acids

Essential fatty acids are great for skin in general and acne in particular. Metabolism of the essential fatty acids (EFAs) in an organism leads to synthesis of eicosanoids, which have various biological properties. Linoleic acid plays an important part in maintaining of healthy skin by prevention of transepidermal water loss[22]. Also, fish oil, which is rich in linoleic acid, and evening primrose oil, which is rich in gamma-linoleic acid, are used in treatment of atopic dermatitis and other skin conditions including acne. EFAs also help in thinning the sebum which clogs the pore.

Our body cannot produce essential fatty acids so we have to take them from outside, from supplements or foods rich in fatty acids. Omega-3 essential fatty acids contain in fatty seafood, especially salmon, and avocados, almonds, wheat germ, soybean and flaxseed oils. Extra virgin olive oil is an excellent source of beneficial fatty acids and polyphenols that have powerful anti-aging action. Organic eggs from free-run farms are an excellent and delicious source of omega-3 acids. And of course, you can find different versions of capsulated Omega-3 supplements in any health food store.

According to recent well-designed (double-blind placebo-controlled randomized cross-over study) study in Belgium, a decrease in linoleic acid in the sebum could be responsible, in part, for acne. When doctors applied linoleic acid topically on the microcomedones in patients with mild acne, they achieved an almost 25% reduction in the overall size of acne eruptions in one month[23]. Today, you can find linoleic acid in such organic topical treatments as Wild Rose Imperfection-Targeting Oil by Korres and Facial Moisture Serum by Suki. You will also consume a lot of essential fatty acids as part of Clear Skin Diet.

Magnesium

Another mineral helpful in improving acne is magnesium. It is essential for metabolism, aids in growth of bones and is the major electrolyte in the body. It is helpful in relieving stress and is responsible for the health of the heart, blood circulation, blood pressure and overall relaxation. Magnesium deficiency is well known to produce mood disorders. A new study shows rapid recovery (less than 7 days) from major depression using 125-300 mg of magnesium (as glycinate and taurinate) with each meal and at bedtime[24]. Magnesium can help in reducing stress, relaxing muscles and thus reducing formation of extra hormones and avoiding acne worsening. Magnesium rich foods are meats, seafood, green vegetable, dairy products, nuts, bananas, peanut butter and potatoes. In the next chapters we will show you how to create simple yet delicious healthy meals using these acne-fighting ingredients.

HOW TO CHOOSE HERBAL SUPPLEMENTS

The use of herbal medicines is common in Europe. In Germany, doctors study herbal therapy in medical school, and a regulatory commission oversees herbal preparations. In North America, on the other hand, herbal medicines are regarded as dietary supplements, and thus not regulated as drugs by the government.

Herbal products as dietary supplements are regulated under the 1994 Dietary Supplement Health and Education Act[25]. FDA does not recognize herbal supplements as a medicine, but they don't acknowledge the effectiveness of herbs. This act ensures that the supplement industry provides consumers with accurate, non-misleading information on dietary supplements. Under this act, supplement manufacturers are not required to perform any tests of product composition, quality, strength, or effectiveness. That's why if the herbal supplement lists any health or benefit claims, the packaging must carry the disclaimer, "This statement has not been evaluated by the Food and Drug Administration. This product is not intended to diagnose, treat, cure, or prevent any disease."

Herbal supplements manufacturers are allowed to make health claims on labels that describe the supplement's effects on general health and well-being or the role of the product in maintaining normal structure and functions of the body. They are strictly prohibited from making disease-related claims which means cannot say that a supplement can treat, prevent, or cure a specific disease.

However, supplement labels can now make claims about common acne, because it is not considered a disease.

Herbal supplements are made of plants, which are a natural substance, and strength of herbal preparations greatly depends on the time of harvest, soil, and storage. With so many manufacturers of herbal supplements, from small businesses to large corporations, there are little guidelines to ensure that all supplements contain the same quantity of active components and are of the same potency. When picking an herbal supplement you should look for the word "standardized" next to the dosage: this means that a supplement has been tested and shown to have a certain amount of the active ingredient in the recommended serving size.

Whichever herb you decide to buy it should come from a pure certified source. Don't buy herbal supplements from companies you know little about. You would want to buy a herb that has not been sprayed with pesticides or other chemicals, and has been harvested and stored in clean hygienic conditions. That's why it's important to buy herbal supplements from a trusted manufacturer that has a solid reputation and is sold in a nationwide drugstore chain.

Many herbs are fairly safe when consumed as directed on package labels. Serious side effects have occurred most commonly when an individual took more than the recommended amount of an herb or mixed supplements with other supplements or prescription drugs. When using supplements, always follow label guidelines for use and dosages. You may choose to seek the guidance of a healthcare practitioner who is familiar with properties of herbs.

If you choose to try a supplement, think of it as an experiment, not a proven medical treatment, and take appropriate precautions. Follow the guidelines in this book. Expect to do some research about specific herbs and different brands of supplements. Be on the lookout for side effects and other problems.

HERBAL SUPPLEMENTS THAT HELP CLEAR THE SKIN

Burdock Root *(Arctium lappa/Arctium minus/Arctium tomentosum)*

Burdock root is the most important herb for treating all forms of chronic skin problems. Burdock root is often described as a "blood purifier", and contributes to clearing the bloodstream of toxins being a mild laxative. Medicinally, burdock root is used both internally and externally for acne, eczema and psoriasis, as well as to treat painful joints and as a diuretic. The herb contains polyacetylenes that have both anti-bacterial and anti-fungal properties. You can find burdock in many detoxifying blends and teas. If you choose to take it as a part of detoxifying course, make sure to check if you are not doubling the intake of other ingredients. Burdock should not be taken by pregnant women as it may cause birth defects and miscarriage.

Chamomile *(Matricaria recutita, Chamaemelum nobile)*

Chamomile both have been used traditionally to calm nerves, to treat various digestive disorders, and to treat a range of skin conditions and mild infections. The medicinal use of chamomile dates back thousands of years to the ancient Egyptians, Romans, and Greeks. Chamomile has been used to treat a variety of conditions including sore throats, gum inflammation (gingivitis), psoriasis, eczema, and acne. While studies in people are few, animal studies have demonstrated German chamomile's ability to reduce inflammation, speed wound healing, reduce muscle spasms, and to serve as a mild sedative to help with relaxation which is also good for your skin. Dried Chamomile flowers can be used to make chamomile tea or mixed with water and applied to acne lesions as a poultice. Chamomile is considered generally safe by the FDA. Because of its calming effects, chamomile should not be taken in conjunction with sedative medications.

Yellow Dock *(Rumex crispus)*

Yellow dock has been known to help improve bladder and liver functions by stimulating bile and digestive enzymes. By this yellow dock reduces bowel inflammation. Yellow dock is also used to treat chronic skin eruptions associated with the toxicity of the intestines. It's extremely powerful against acne! Yellow dock has a mild laxative effect, due to component called anthraquinone glycoside. Yellow dock may cause mild diarrhea in some people. Don't use yellow dock if you are pregnant or nursing.

Milk Thistle *(Silybum marianum)*

Milk Thistle has been used since Greco-Roman times as an herbal remedy for liver problems as liver and kidney tonic and digestive aid. The active substance, silymarin, is known to protect liver against many chemical toxins, and increase the healthy function and regeneration of this vital organ. Milk thistle helps cleanse, detoxify, rebuild and restore healthy liver function. Poor liver operation results in improper waste elimination, which leads to skin eruptions and acne.

Preliminary laboratory studies even suggest that milk thistle may have anti-cancer effects. Most milk thistle products are standardized preparations that are easy to use. Side effects from milk thistle are very uncommon, but may include stomach pain, nausea, vomiting, diarrhea, headache, or rash. Milk thistle should not be used by pregnant or breastfeeding women.

Black Cohosh (*Actaea racemosa*)

Black Cohosh has been used as a healing herb by Native Americans for centuries. Black Cohosh root extract is most famous for its ability to relieve the symptoms commonly associated with to alleviate the symptoms of PMS and menopause[27]. Gently regulating your hormones with herbal supplements will result in great diminishing of acne outbreaks by itself. There is also some evidence to suggest that Black Cohosh helps alleviate depression, and that it has anti-inflammatory properties. Controversy remains regarding the safety of Black Cohosh in women with a personal history or strong family history of breast cancer[28]. Consult your physician before taking this herb because it's quote potent. Black Cohosh should be avoided during pregnancy and during nursing.

Kampo

A few reports have shown that Japanese Kampo herbal supplement Keigai-rengyo-to (TJ-50) may be effective in the treatment of acne. Researchers suggest that Kampo improves the skin condition thanks to its antibacterial and anti-inflammatory properties. Kampo formulation contains seventeen herbs, including Skullcap root (Scutellaria lateriflora), licorice root (Glycyrrhiza glabra), mint (Mentha arvensis), Angelica root (Angelica archangelica), peony root (Paeonia lactiflora) and many others[29].

Ayurveda

Ayurveda, an ancient Indian holistic alternative medicine, classifies patients by body types, or prakriti, which are determined by proportions of the three doshas, or body zones. Ayurveda considers acne as an aggravation of Pitta dosha. The treatment includes a diet that includes plenty of bland foods such as oatmeal, apple sauce, basmati rice and eliminating fried foods, spicy foods and citrus fruits, and an herbal supplement intake. This practice is well-documented for its effectiveness. In one reliable trial, people with moderate acne were randomly assigned to receive either placebo or different Ayurvedic preparations. Only one formulation, Sunder Vati, significantly reduced the number and severity of inflamed acne lesions. Non-inflammatory lesions were also reduced and more than 65% of patients on Sunder Vati showed improvement in overall facial acne condition. All the preparations were well-tolerated[30]. The herbs in the Sunder Vati preparation include Ginger (Zingiber officinale), Holarrhena antidysenterica, and Embelia ribes among others.

Homeopathy

As a holistic treatment, homeopathy looks at the body as a whole, inside and outside. Homeopathy considers acne to be a sign of an underlying health condition. Professional homeopaths may recommend one or more of the following treatments for acne after studying your physical, emotional, and intellectual health. The following compositions are most commonly prescribed for acne:

Calendula topical ointments for skin conditions involving pustules or inflamed lesions;

Hepar sulphur for severe inflammatory acne;

Kali bromatum for moderate to severe hormonal acne, especially on the forehead;

Silicea for whiteheads and excessive sweating.

CLEAR SKIN DIET

Almost all authors who write about acne claim that food by itself doesn't cause acne. In every article about acne and almost every book about beauty in chapter titled "Acne Myths" you will read that eating chocolate, fries, candy, cakes, buns and fast food makes no impact on acne. This sounds comforting to most readers, as they learn later that the key to their success in defeating acne is lots and lots of benzoyl peroxide. Eat your doughnuts and apply some more BP! Except for two poorly designed studies, now more than 30 years old, there are few objective data to support the notion that food and acne are not linked.[31]

In contrast, more and more doctors today believe that there is a close connection between diet and acne. A large body of evidence now exists showing how diet may directly or indirectly influence the following causes of acne, starting with increased production of skin cells in the skin pore, followed by the pore blockage, the colonization of the comedo by P. acnes bacteria, and the inflammation both within the pimple and in the area around it.

Today, diet remains the third most frequently implicated factor (after hormones and genetics) as the cause of the disease, with 32% of the respondents selecting diet as the main cause, and 44% thinking that foods aggravate acne.[32] In another study that questioned knowledge about causes of acne among English teenagers, 11% of the responders blamed greasy food as the main cause of the disease, whereas in another study found that 41% of final-year medical students of the University of Melbourne chose diet as an important factor of acne flare-ups[33].

We are what we eat, and the skin reflects what's going on inside our body. If we eat lots of fruits and vegetables, consume yoghurt and lean meats, we have healthy skin, hair and lean muscle. That's common sense. If we eat junk food, we have pimples, cellulite and generally, what Bridget Jones called, "blobby bits" all over the body.

The energy that we get from foods comes from three types of nutrients: fats, proteins, and carbohydrates. When foods are digested, they are broken down into the body's basic fuel glucose, a type of sugar. The glucose is absorbed by the bloodstream, and is then known as blood glucose or blood sugar. Any food will raise blood sugar to some extent[34] but different foods are converted to sugar at different speed. Fats need up to six to eight or more hours after a meal to be converted into glucose. Protein such as meats, poultry, fish, eggs, and soy need about three to four hours after a meal to convert into blood glucose. Carbohydrates, such as sugars and starches, are rapidly turned into blood glucose causing a spike in insulin production.

All the sweet and starchy foods—including starches such as rice, pasta, breads, cereals, and similar foods; fruits and juices; milk and milk products; and anything made with added sugars, such as candies, cookies, cakes, and pies—are easily converted into sugar by enzymes in our digestive system. Candy, sweets, cookies, pasta, breads—all they make the blood sugar raise, which makes us feel a short but intense burst of energy.

If we eat foods that cause stress to our body by raising the level of stress-inducing blood sugar, we increase inflammation and oiliness in skin. Why does it happen? Refined carbohydrates and sugar lead to a surge of insulin and an insulin-like growth factor called IGF-1 in your body. This can lead to an excess of male hormones, which cause pores in the skin to secrete sebum more actively. The pore stretches, breaks, oil and bacteria build up. The acne lesion is born.

Chemical reactions caused by sugar are the number one cause of acne, and the worse the acne the more likely sugar is involved. Eating a sugar-rich food to which the body is addicted (and we are truly addicted to sugar, consuming it in high doses all our lives) leads to a continuous over-abundance of insulin and as a result, over-production of sebum. In such a case the immune system fights the food as if it were an invading organism. This can cause inflammation in the skin (and many other conditions), as well as the need to eliminate the toxin.

There is another link between food and acne that is scientifically proven. The male hormone, testosterone, stimulates the production of the sebaceous glands in times of stress. Meat contains hormones and hormone-like substances which can affect the hormonal balance in the body. Dermatologists have reported that women who regularly eat meat are more likely to suffer from acne and hirsutism (the excessive growth of thick dark hair in locations where hair growth in women usually is minimal or absent) which they put down to the steroids and hormone levels in the meat.[35]

WHAT TO EAT IF YOU WANT TO HAVE ACNE

Let's take a look at the typical all-American diet. For breakfast, you eat a white toast with butter, an egg or two fried together with crispy bacon, and a cup of coffee. For lunch, you most likely have a roast beef, meat ball, or chicken sandwich with French fries on side, and a soft drink. When afternoon snack time comes, you have a bag of potato chips, a candy bar, or maybe a doughnut. For dinner, you will have a feast of a pork chop, a fish fried in batter, or another burger with mashed potatoes, fries, or in better cases, a salad with ranch dressing. To top the day, you treat yourself to hearty portion of ice cream or an apple pie.

All day long, you are consuming fats and sugars in quantities sufficient enough to feed a town in third world country. Baked and fried foods such as burgers, hams, roast beef, chicken strips, fish and chips, and pork chops are overloaded with trans (hydrogenated) fats which cause excessive production of proinflammatory cytokines leading to acne[35]. White bread in toasts and sandwiches, ice cream, apple pies, and candy bars are converted to sugar at a rapid rate causing spikes in insulin levels, increasing the level of sebum production and promoting the inflammation in your skin. No wonder your skin looks greasy, shiny, and inflamed, lacking tone and healthy glow.

Of course not all people who eat burgers and fries on a daily basis have acne. But if you already have acne, revising your bad eating habits can dramatically improve the look of your skin. It may not be easy. Fast foods are convenient; apple pies and ice cream bring instant comfort and positive emotions when you are feeling down, while burgers and meatloaf in gravy are staples of many traditional family dinners.

We don't expect you to make a life-long commitment and cancel delicious foods from your menu forever. Instead, take a small step and try eating anti-acne diet rich in vitamins, protein, fiber, good carbs, and essential fatty acids for just one month. By controlling your sugar and fat intake while adding essential fatty acids and good proteins you will day by day clear your skin from within. And when you see the clear difference, you will know that you are doing well for your body, as skin is a clear reflection of what's going on inside of you.

FORBIDDEN FRUITS (AND OTHER FOODS)

During Clear Skin Diet we will be avoiding foods that promote inflammation on cellular level and increase the production of sebum. The easiest way to tell the good food from the bad food is using the glycemic index, which is well-known to people with diabetes. Proteins such as lean non-red meat, seafood, beans, non-saturated fats and most vegetables have low glycemic rating. That means they are less likely to cause a hike in the blood sugar level. Potatoes, pasta, rice, cakes, cookies, sweets of all kinds have high glycemic level.

First of all, we will avoid any foods that contain processed starch and sugars. This includes all kinds of bread, well-cooked pasta, noodles, rice, cookies, muffins, doughnuts, crackers, boxed cereals (except for steel-cut and rolled cereals that require cooking.) Say good-bye to pizza, hot dogs and burgers—if you already didn't. However, you may still eat low-fat pizza on whole grain crust and lean meat sandwiches on whole wheat bread.

Sugar is the major no-no if you have acne. We all know that sugary foods are bad for our looks, and now we know why. Even though they give you an energy boost, highly sugared foods are proven to reduce your body's ability to fight off infection. There is medical evidence that ingesting just 100 grams of sugar in any form—be it glucose, fructose, sucrose, honey or orange juice from concentrate—can reduce your immune system's ability to function by as much as 50 per cent. This effect can last for up to five hours. And since we consume much more than 100 g of sugar every day, the effect can be very long-lasting. What does it mean? While healthy immune system can heal a pimple in 5-7 days, an immune system weakened by sugar intake will not be able to fight the inflammation in the zit, and it may ripen for the whole ten days or even two weeks, most likely leaving an ugly mark behind[36].

Another group of foods to avoid if you have acne is vegetables and fruits rich in starch. This includes potatoes, mango, bananas, and melons. Don't you notice similarities in their "floury" texture? Besides, tropical fruits are sweeter than domestic fruits. Apples, pears, peaches, plums and berries are considered domestic fruits and are all acceptable.

There are some restrictions in the dessert area, too. During Clear Skin Diet you will avoid ice creams including sherbet, frozen yoghurt and milkshakes. Same refers to jams, pudding, marmalades, jellies and syrups. The only desserts you should get used to are fruit salads and fruit cocktails made *without* tropical fruits or melons.

Whether fruit juices are natural or made from concentrate, they all contain large amounts of simple sugars. Natural fruit juices are OK, but you should avoid those with refined sugars. Instead, try making your own juice from carrots, beets or celery (dilute half-and-half with purified water). Add a little fresh ginger root to 'spice' things up!

If you are a regular coffee drinker, you may still have a small amount of coffee during this program (max. two cups daily). Large amounts of coffee weaken the immune system and place additional stress upon the adrenal glands. Herbal and green teas are acceptable. It is strongly recommended to not consume alcohol of any type during this diet.

You may ask, why do we have to stay away from "good" foods that are mainstay of many other popular diets? What's so bad about bananas, fruit juices or cereal? All foods are converted into sugars by enzymes in our digestive system. Even if the food is not clearly "sugary", it may be quickly converted into sugar causing the unwanted rise in blood sugar—and we already know the consequences.

To help you pick the food healthiest for your skin you may use Glycemic Index initially developed for people with diabetes. Available online at www. glycemicindex.com, this helpful service rates all foods on the glycemic index, ranging from water (which is zero) to pure sugar (GI 100). This difference shows the impact the food has on the blood sugar level. You simply enter the name of the food, and the system provides you with glycemic index of all meals that contain this product. For example, raw apple has glycemic index of 34, while apple muffin has GI of 44. To help clear your skin you should avoid any food that has glycemic index over 40. In the next chapter we will introduce you to the Clear Acne Diet that contain delicious healthy recipes that contain fats, carbohydrates, and proteins at each meal at an appropriate calorie level to both provide essential nutrients and create an steady level of blood glucose during the day. Eating blood-friendly foods is easy, and soon you will be able to recognize acne-provoking foods at glance and form your eating habits accordingly.

Amazingly similar approach to acne diet we can find in traditional Chinese medicine, where each food is claimed to have different energetic qualities. People with acne should avoid consuming foods that are "warming" and "damp" and instead consume foods that are "cooling" and rich in water. Warming and sticky foods, such as deep-fried foods, meat, sugar, chocolate and alcohol, are hard to digest. Cooling water-rich foods, such as cucumbers, carrots, celery, lettuce, cabbage, beet, pears, cherries, papaya, and watermelon, help cool the blood, decrease toxins and improve digestion.

According to Isaac Asimov, Russian-born biochemist and science fiction writer, the first law of dietetics states: "If it tastes good, it's bad for you." Today, thanks to the fabulous variety of healthy mouth-watering food choices in grocery stores and the abundance of health food stores and organic markets we don't need to limit our choices when it comes to picking low-starch, low-sugar food that would be good for our skin. By following this dietary approach you will improve liver function and bowel movements, helping intestines to eliminate toxins and clear skin from inside.

CLEAR SKIN DIET INGREDIENTS

We have designed a simple, delicious, fun, and affordable diet that improves the condition of your skin effectively and without any side effects. In matter of days your acne will start to heal faster, your skin tone will become glowing and radiant, and even some extra inches around your hips and waist will begin to slowly but steadily disappear.

This diet is based around lots of vegetables, fruits and good protein rich in essential fatty acids and poor in cholesterol. We will also eat foods that help the body cleanse itself more efficiently by eliminating toxins and other waste. Each meal will contain proteins, low-glycemic carbohydrates and essential fatty acids that keep you energized for hours.

Intensely colored vegetables such as arugula, artichokes, asparagus, green beans, beets or beet tops, Bok Choy, broccoli, Brussels sprouts, cabbage, carrots, celery, collards, chards, cucumbers, dandelion, endive, escarole, kale, kohlrabi, lettuce, parsley, parsnips, radishes, scallions, spinach, zucchini, watercress are all great. Even though it's mainly white, cauliflower is not the food to be overlooked. All these vegetables have the lowest impact on your blood sugar, and, therefore, should form the basis of the healthy anti-acne diet.

Herbs for seasoning, such as basil, oregano, thyme, coriander, are welcome in the diet. Mushrooms are also allowed, except shitake mushroom for its high glycemic index. Olives are also allowed, canned or marinated, black and green. Vegetables may be cooked (lightly steamed is preferable) or eaten raw. Apples, berries, currants, grapes, apricots, prunes, peaches, plums, nectarines and cherries will make a delicious addition to your anti-acne diet. Feel free to eat them as much as you like.

Proteins

Good source of protein, such as low-fat chicken, turkey, dairy, veal, soy substitutes, and fish are the basis of your breakfast, lunch, and dinner. This way, you stay energized and full throughout the day and will not fall prey of mid-afternoon fast-food cravings.

Essential fatty acids

Essential fatty acids are important part of Clear Skin Diet. Research published in the Journal of American Academy of Dermatology has shown that essential fatty acids (EFA) can help with hormonal imbalances that lead to acne. In fact, people with hormonal related acne have been shown to have deficiencies of Essential Fatty Acids. Extra virgin olive oil, grapeseed oil, flaxseed and flaxseed oil are all good sources of alpha-linolenic acid (ALA), the plant-based omega-3 A quarter-cup (1 ounce) of walnuts or almonds supplies about 2 grams of plant-based omega-3 fatty acids, slightly more than is found in 3 ounces of salmon. Pumpkin seeds and walnuts are great sources of omega-3 fatty acids, too.

Venison and buffalo are both good sources of both omega-3 acid and protein. These wild game meats can be purchased through mail-order sources if your local groceries don't carry them. For vegetarians, soy beans and tofu are excellent sources of protein. Try rice protein or whey or egg protein if you are a lacto-vegetarian.

Although the best source of essential fatty acids would be salmon, we do not recommend eating it more than two times a week, because most often the salmon you find in your grocery stores may be contaminated with mercury, and organically grown salmon is quite costly for daily use. Still, when you feel like eating fish for lunch or dinner, buy salmon that was fished, not farmed, or better yet, certified organic salmon from a trustworthy supplier. Other fatty, preferably cold-water fish, including herring (both Atlantic and Pacific), sardines, Atlantic halibut, bluefish, tuna, and Atlantic mackerel are all good substitutes for salmon. The mineral iodine, in high dietary levels, can contribute to acne causing pores to swell, leading to acne breakouts. To reduce your iodine intake, avoid iodized salt, shrimp, and sea vegetables.

Drinks

There has been a suggestion that dairy aggravates acne. Milk contains two proteins; casein and whey. Casein gives much of the allergy problems associated with milk, whereas whey has demonstrated immunological stimulating properties. Therefore, you may continue consuming milk in moderation, but only in lactose-free non-fat versions.

Green tea, water-diluted fruit juices, tomato juice, and plain non-carbonated water are the only drinks permitted during the Clear Skin Diet. When you buy tomato juice, stick to plain juice without spices and MSG. The best tomato juice is made by Hanes (the makers of ketchup) or by your local manufacturers.

Another drink that greatly improves the condition of your skin is probiotic drink such as plain yogurt, kefir, or ayran. The dietary use of probiotics has a long history. The use of microorganisms to produce and preserve the food is known for millenniums. The Bible and the sacred books of Hinduism mention the common use of sour dairy products centuries ago. Fermented milk drinks, such as kefir, kumis, ayran, lassi, kombucha and other dairy products were often used therapeutically before the existence of microorganisms was recognized. These drinks are dietary staples in many countries.

Probiotics are live microorganisms as food supplement in order to benefit health. They help clear skin conditions thanks to the general cleansing action of the friendly bacteria 61. In 1964, Dr. R.H. Siver in a paper entitled "Lactobacillus for the Control of Acne" reported the 80% improvement of acne in 300 patients treated with the eight-day course of a lactic bacterium combination. A more recent German study has shown that bifidobacteria intake improves the severe atopic eczema[37].

Probiotics are available as nutritional supplements and in functional foods, such as yogurts, are most commonly the Bifidobacterium species and the Lactobacillus species. We have found an interesting suggestion on applying probiotics topically. Take a caplet of a probiotic formulation and mix the powder with distilled water to form a smooth paste. After washing your face, apply the probiotic paste to the area where acne erupts most often. Leave the paste on for twenty minutes or longer before rinsing it off gently with warm water. In addition to helping clear up acne, this paste helps lighten acne marks thanks to the gentle exfoliating action of lactic acid.

Probiotics are generally well tolerated, but if you take too much, you may end up with constipation. By gradually increasing the intake of Bifidobacterium species you will have a regular healthy painless bowel movement. In a few pages you will learn how to make a probiotic-rich healthy drink at home spending very little money.

In general, Clear Skin Diet is comprised of five meals each divided by three hours. We encourage you to follow this diet for twenty-one day to see visible results. Why twenty-one day? Studies show that it's exactly how much time an average person needs to build a strong habit. Twenty-one day later, if you scrupulously follow the diet, you will form new clear skin—and clear body!—eating habits. You will be able to instantly pick foods that are good for your skin, and you will be able to experiment with new meals based on Clear Skin Diet principles, so that you will never feel deprived or bored.

Nothing feels better than sweet taste of success and Clear Skin Diet does just that, of course, if you don't cut corners and cheat.

10-DAY SAMPLE EATING PLAN

Before starting the plan, make sure you have all ingredients you need for just three days. It's best to eat the freshest possible food. Make a smart grocery shopping list: buy pre-cooked chicken and turkey breast, organic salmon filets, veal cutlets, and gentle berries and grapes just in quantity enough to fit in your diet plan, while water, apples, pears, grapefruits, and other sturdy fruit can be bought in bulk. Scout your pantry, fridge, and kitchen cabinets for stray packs of crackers, candies, snack foods, and ice cream. Explain your family members that you are going on a diet, and encourage them to join you, or cook smaller meals for yourself and let them indulge in their favourite foods. When they see how great you look, they will beg you to cook these delicious meals for them, too!

You will notice that daily food plans are quite similar. You don't have to follow the day by day in exact same order. If you feel like cooking chicken breast on Day Two instead of turkey sandwich, go for it. The only important thing is to swap the whole day's menu altogether, because all meals during the day are designed to work in sync. A nutritious daily menu should contain proteins and whole grains, vegetables and fruit for fibre, vitamins, and antioxidants such as skin-clarifying lycopen in watermelons. All the meals in the diet plan are unique and full of flavor, so there's little chance the boredom gets you down.

If you don't have skin-friendly food choices for lunch at work, prepare the lunch and afternoon snack the evening before. When you plan ahead your meals you are less likely to grab a slice of pizza or doughnut. Set aside leftovers for your lunch when preparing dinner, and take half-hour off your weekend to chop fruits and vegetables for fruit and side salads and pack them in resealable bags. Pack the lunch of your day and store it in the fridge if it contains more delicate ingredients such as strawberries or watermelon. Buy spring bottled water in large packs (24 and up) preferably in glass bottles and low-fat milk in large cartons. Health food stores have the best selection of organic green and herbal teas, and they usually cost less than similar brands in supermarkets. Use these smart tricks, and your skin (and wallet) will thank you.

DAY ONE

Wake Up
½ liter of spring/purified water with 1 tbsp of apple cider vinegar

Breakfast
Omelet made of two egg whites and one whole egg with chopped spinach and red bell peppers
Plain low-fat yogurt or homemade kefir
Green tea, rooibos or mate with honey if desired.

Lunch
Grilled chicken sandwich: sliced grilled chicken breast sprinkled with virgin olive oil, tomatoes, mesclun greens, Romano lettuce, and green bell peppers on whole wheat bread
Fruit salad: blueberries, strawberries, watermelon chunks, grapes, and chopped almonds

Afternoon snack
1 sliced tomato with 25g feta cheese and 3 olives
Green tea, rooibos or mate

Dinner
Oven-barbequed turkey breast marinated in honey, soy sauce and red pepper sauce
Romaine lettuce, apple, goat's cheese and carrot salad seasoned with olive oil and lemon juice
Herbal tea: chamomile, valerian or Melissa blend with honey if desired

Bedtime snack
2 sliced apples with organic honey

DAY TWO

Wake Up
½ liter of spring/purified water with 1 tbsp of apple cider vinegar

Breakfast
Steel-cut oatmeal topped with blueberries, strawberries, and chopped almonds
Plain low-fat yogurt or homemade kefir
Green tea, rooibos or mate with honey if desired

Lunch

Maple turkey breast and snow peas salad with mixed greens: Romaine lettuce, alfa alfa sprouts, broccoli florets, spinach, and watercress seasoned with olive oil and lemon juice

Fruit salad: apples, pears, watermelon and two dates

Afternoon snack

Large sushi roll made of brown rice and salmon with pickled ginger

Green tea

Dinner

Pan-fried 2 oz salmon filet (palm-sized) seasoned with lemon juice

Low-fat cole slaw: shredded cabbage, shredded carrot, 1 tbsp chopped parsley, seasoned with Dijon mustard, lemon juice and virgin olive oil

Herbal tea: chamomile, valerian or melissa blend with honey if desired

Bedtime snack

Dried dates, raisins and apple topped with honey

DAY THREE

Wake Up

½ liter of spring/purified water with 1 tbsp of apple cider vinegar

Breakfast

French toast made of whole wheat bread dipped in beaten egg and sprinkled with oil from orange zest, then fried on 1/2 tsp of olive oil

Plain low-fat yogurt or kefir

A handful of mixed berries

Green tea, rooibos or mate with honey if desired

Lunch

Medium bowl of salad made of Romaine lettuce, grape tomatoes, spinach, celery, apple and chopped almond, topped with 2 oz low-fat grilled chicken

2 pears

Afternoon snack

Rye bread snaps dipped into 2 tbsp low-fat tzatziki dipping sauce (cucumber, peppermint and plain yogurt mix)

Green tea, rooibos or mate

Dinner
1 grilled eggplant topped with feta cheese and chopped parsley
Fresh mussel and shrimp salad with green beans, red and yellow pepper, black olives and Romaine lettuce, topped with olive oil, black pepper and lemon juice
Herbal tea: chamomile, valerian or melissa blend with honey if desired to calm down your nerves.

Bedtime snack
An apple and a pear

DAY FOUR

Wake Up
½ liter of spring/purified water with 1 tbsp of apple cider vinegar

Breakfast
1 whole wheat bagel with organic low-fat cream cheese
1 boiled egg or egg Benedictine without sauce
Plain low-fat yogurt or kefir
Green tea, rooibos or mate with honey if desired.

Lunch
Hot chicken salad: sliced roasted chicken breast, Romaine lettuce, arugula, sweet onions, spinach, radicchio, and toasted pine nuts, dressed with raspberry wine vinegar and virgin olive oil
Skim-milk mozzarella stick

Afternoon snack
Toasted whole wheat bagel with hummus
Baby carrots and celery sticks, as many as you like
Green tea, rooibos or mate

Dinner
Oven-baked turkey sautéed in orange juice and sprinkled with almonds
Spring salad: Romaine lettuce, arugula, fresh mushrooms and radishes dressed with juice of one lemon

Herbal tea: chamomile, valerian or melissa blend with honey if desired to calm down your nerves.

Bedtime snack
Toasted almonds with honey

DAY FIVE

Wake Up
½ liter of spring/purified water with 1 tbsp of apple cider vinegar

Breakfast
Rice with dates: add 5 sliced dates when rice is half-cooked
Plain low-fat yogurt or kefir
Green tea, rooibos or mate with honey if desired.

Lunch
Chicken quesadilla sandwich: whole wheat tortilla filled with sliced chicken breast, chopped fresh cilantro, olives, Romaine lettuce, shredded skim-milk mozzarella cheese and chopped green chillies to taste. Season with salsa if desired.
Fruit salad: blueberries, strawberries, blackberries, and pineapple

Afternoon snack
Instant miso soup
Edamame (soy) beans dipped in hummus
Green tea

Dinner
6-7 pan-fried scallops, sprinkled with chopped rosemary
Green salad with gruyere cheese: Romaine lettuce, zucchini, endives, one hard-boiled egg topped with 2 tbsp of grated gruyere or Emmentaler cheese and juice of ½ lemon
Herbal tea: chamomile, valerian or Melissa blend with honey if desired to calm down your nerves.

Bedtime snack
1 cup of low-fat cottage cheese topped with 1 sliced peach

DAY SIX

Wake Up
½ liter of spring/purified water with 1 tbsp of apple cider vinegar

Breakfast
1 cup of bran sugar-free cereal topped with ½ cup of blueberries, low-fat yogurt or kefir
1 soft boiled egg
Green tea, rooibos or mate with honey if desired.

Lunch
Smoked salmon sandwich: 3 oz smoken salmon, 3 sliced cherry tomatoes, Romaine lettuce, 2 slices of smoked turkey breast on top of whole wheat roll dressed with low-fat honey mustard.
Fruit salad: gooseberries, blueberries, raspberries, sliced peach

Afternoon snack
1 cup of strawberries topped with low-fat whipped cream

Dinner
Grilled chicken breast, seasoned with rosemary, basil and black pepper
Tossed green salad with grated carrot: toss watercress, chicory, 1 apple, 1 grated carrot, and dress with low-fat Ranch dressing
Herbal tea: chamomile or valerian blend with honey if desired to calm down your nerves.

Bedtime snack
1 cup frozen low-fat yogurt topped with blueberries

DAY SEVEN

Wake Up
½ liter of spring/purified water with 1 tbsp of apple cider vinegar

Breakfast
Omelet made of two whole eggs, chopped parsley, spinach and mushrooms
Plain yogurt or homemade kefir
Green tea, rooibos or mate with honey if desired.

Lunch
Whole wheat pasta salad: cooked pasta mixed with ¼ cup sun-dried tomatoes, 2 cooked artichoke hearts, chopped basil and 3 oz (100g) sliced chicken breast. Season with balsamic vinegar if desired.
Fruit salad: watermelon, honeydew, pineapple and blueberries

Afternoon snack
Half whole wheat English muffin topped with low-fat organic cream cheese and smoken salmon

Dinner
Salad Nicoise: Romaine lettuce, green beans, bell peppers, tomatoes, small red onion, anchovy fillets, 2 oz tuna chunks, 2 hard-boiled eggs dressed with lemon juice
Herbal tea: chamomile, valerian or melissa blend with honey if desired to calm down your nerves.

Bedtime snack
Skim ricotta cheese and honey spread over half of small whole wheat bagel

DAY EIGHT

Wake Up
½ liter of spring/purified water with 1 tbsp of apple cider vinegar

Breakfast
Sliced honeydew melon, pear and peach mixed with steel-cut cooked oatmeal
Plain yogurt or homemade kefir
Green tea, rooibos or mate with honey if desired.

Lunch
Warm green chicken liver salad: pre-cooked chicken livers, Romaine lettuce, arugula, spinach, cauliflower florets, chopped fresh chives, dressed with balsamic vinegar and pepper
2 apples

Afternoon snack

Tomato mozzarella sandwich: 1 sliced tomato, mozzarella, basil leaves arranged on top of whole wheat toast, sprinkled with virgin olive oil

Dinner

Mussel and salmon salad: 2 oz pan-fried salmon cut in chunks, 5 large New Zealand mussels mixed in bowl with green beans, yellow green pepper, pitted black olives, arugula, watercress, and dressed with lemon juice and pepper.

Strawberry and orange compote: 1 cup strawberries cooked in 1/2 cup orange juice for 20 min or until thick.

Herbal tea: chamomile, valerian or melissa blend with honey if desired to calm down your nerves.

Bedtime snack

2 instant blueberry buckwheat pancakes topped with honey

DAY NINE

Wake Up

½ liter of spring/purified water with 1 tbsp of apple cider vinegar

Breakfast

Whole bread toast with skim-milk melted mozzarella
2 scrambled eggs
Plain yogurt or homemade kefir
Green tea, rooibos or mate with honey if desired.

Lunch

Easy salmon salad: 2 oz smoked salmon, 1 celery stalk, 1 hard-boiled egg, Romaine lettuce mixed and dressed with virgin olive oil and lemon juice

Fruit salad: blueberries, gooseberries, apple, pear, peach with 1 tsp honey

Afternoon snack

Whole wheat bagel toasted and topped with 1 tsp low-fat peanut butter and sliced apple

Dinner

Gremolada turkey: ½ lbs turkey breast baked in oven and topped with Gremolada: ½ cup chopped parsley minced with 1 clove of garlic and 1 tsp grated lemon peel.

Tossed green salad: small head of Romaine lettuce, Belgian endives, ½ head radicchio salad, chopped and dressed with virgin olive oil and chopped basil.

Herbal tea: chamomile, valerian or Melissa blend with honey if desired to calm down your nerves.

Bedtime snack

2 low-fat waffles topped with blueberries and honey

DAY TEN

Wake Up

½ liter of spring/purified water with 1 tbsp of apple cider vinegar

Breakfast

Stuff ¼ cup leftover turkey or chicken mixed with 1 sliced green pepper and 1 oz grated skim milk mozzarella cheese into whole wheat pita bread. Toast until cheese melts.

Plain yogurt or homemade kefir

Green tea, rooibos or mate with honey if desired.

Lunch

Chicken chef's salad: ½ head Romaine lettuce, 1 red onion (optional), cucumber, 1 hard-boiled egg, 1 sliced radish mixed with cooked chicken strips and dressed with virgin olive oil and lemon juice

Whole wheat crusty roll with hummus

Afternoon snack

Fruit salad: strawberries, peaches, blueberries, watermelon with honey on top

Dinner

Yogurt-lime marinated salmon: 3 oz salmon steak marinated in the mix of plain low-fat yogurt, honey, and chopped garlic. Pan-fry in virgin olive oil with lime wedges on side.

Roquefort salad: 1 head of Romaine lettuce, ½ cup arugula, ½ cup watercress tossed with crumbled Roquefort cheese and dressed with lemon juice and 3 drops of Worcestershire sauce

Herbal tea: chamomile, valerian or Melissa blend with honey if desired to calm down your nerves.

Bedtime snack
Oven-baked apple topped with honey and low-fat whipped cream

This diet is anything but boring. Raw vegetables, fruit and simply cooked meats and fish have comprised human diet for centuries. When at first the amounts of food and the limitation of your protein choices may leave you feeling deprived, remember: over 75% of the world's population have daily menus similar to the Clear Skin Diet, and many more would consider a daily menu like this a feast. And people outside of industrialized countries rarely suffer from acne. Only when they come to Western countries and switch to Western diets, their acne starts to bloom. Experiment with wholesome foods and exotic spices, try new green vegetables and treat yourself with an occasional tropical fruit instead of a cake, and you will never need to treat your acne with antibiotics and retinoids again!

HOW TO PREPARE YOUR OWN PROBIOTIC DRINK

Kefir, a jelly drink resembling thin yogurt, is a traditional probiotic drink for many European cultures. It's often called "milk champagne" due to its bubbly effect and zesty taste. Kefir is perhaps the most potent and vitamin-infused of all probiotic drinks, as it's made of live bacteria and yeast. These bacteria will repopulate in your digestive tract, while yogurt bacteria won't. Besides, milk proteins in kefir are broken down during the fermentation, which makes kefir suitable even for people with lactose intolerance.

Making kefir at home is quite easy and it's cheaper than buying a yogurt. All you need is enough milk and a kefir bacterial culture. When made at home, kefir is free from artificial aromas and preservatives, and you can pick yourself what kind of milk you want to use: organic and low-fat cow milk, or even sheep and goat milk. You can also add some fruit to your kefir and blend it into a smoothie. This delicious complete breakfast drink will do wonders for your complexion.

You can buy kefir bacterial culture in a kefir making kit. All you need is bacterial culture and several 1 liter glass jars with lids. First, you will make a starter by mixing a kefir bacterial culture with 1 liter of milk of your choice. Let it ferment in a room temperature for one day. As soon as the milk thickens forming a jelly with distinctive sour taste, the initial batch of your kefir is ready. To make the next batch, just add 3-4 tbs of this initial batch to 1 liter of warm milk. Keep the remaining initial batch in a refrigerator. As soon as you feel confident, you may experiment with the taste making kefir more or less sour.

Keep your kefir out of direct sunlight in a cool cupboard or in a lowest shelve of your refrigerator. If the jar lid fits too tightly, the buildup of a carbon dioxide gas during the fermentation will cause a bulging "champagne effect" and a loud pop when you open the jar. Avoid using metal spoons when transferring initial batches of kefir to the fresh milk.

If you keep your kefir fermenting longer than usual, you will end up with a double-layer layer liquid: a milk protein on top and whey on bottom. You can use curdled milk to prepare homemade cheese. In some cultures homemade cottage cheese is prepared by boiling the curdled milk in whey until it hardens, then straining it. There's also a simple way: just strain the curdled cheese separating it from whey and leave it in a fridge for one more day. You can use whey to rinse your hair and washing your face. The homemade cottage cheese is an excellent source of protein. You can add it to your salads or eat straight with fruits and honey.

CLEAR SKIN DIET GUIDELINES

Always make sure your meal consists of proteins, low-glycemic (not sweet) carbohydrates and non-saturated fats. **Eat your protein first**, followed by vegetables and fruit and vegetable juices. Eat proteins, such as fish, chicken, lean beef, turkey, sparingly even if they are low-fat. Protein-rich foods can easily increase the blood-protein level, since blood protein level can fluctuate very much. Too high blood protein level can elevate the protein level in the skin, making it temporarily retain more water, pinching off sebum canals.

Replace refined foods, such as white flour, with whole grains. For example, cut down on white bread, pasta made with white flour, and desserts. Whole grains are far more nutritious and provide fiber necessary for optimal colon health. We recommend that you use organic foods as much as possible for this diet.

Measure your portions. Divide you plate in quarters. Proteins must occupy ¼, grains of your choice should fit into another quarter, and the remaining half of the plate must be covered with vegetables, raw or lightly steamed. If you choose to skip grains or proteins, fill in the remaining space with nutritious veggies, such as green beans and broccoli.

Drink a lot of water. Eight cups a day is recommended for flushing toxins out of your body and reducing hunger. Load on antioxidants which can be found in tea, chocolate, red wine, grape juice, herbs and vegetables.

Avoid stimulants, such as coffee or other caffeinated beverages. If you can't function without coffee or tea, indulge in the morning and switch to decaffeinated drinks later in the day. Switch to green tea which has amazing anti-inflammatory benefits. Try drinking it instead of coffee or black tea. Green tea has lower levels of caffeine, and it's delicious and refreshing when iced. Sugared drinks have no nutritional value and provide excess calories. It's best to avoid all these sweet drinks and stick to water.

Keep **healthy snacks** available at home and work. No doubt a fruit makes a healthy snack but according to the latest study, a piece of fruit or some nuts in the midday will make you hungry faster. Researchers at the University of Buffalo in New York found that when people have a mini-meal such as whole wheat bread with slice of lean chicken or tuna salad they don't have cravings for traditional snacks such as crackers or chips. This happens because mini-meals are perceived as a real meal, only smaller.

Eat out right. Managing acne does not have to mean giving up favorite foods, sweets, or restaurants and healthier fast foods such as sushi and Thai. For example, you can always pick a mixed green salad with turkey or chicken for lunch and top it with a portion of fruit salad.

Drink enough water. Either pure spring water or purified water is recommended. We recommend that you drink more than just when you are feeling thirsty. Make it a rule to drink a glass of water (half a ½ liter bottle) every hour. Water will help to flush toxins from your body, especially while you are cleansing.

This diet is not intended for use during pregnancy or breast-feeding, and it's not for children under 12.

ACNE DETOX

We all know that acne pimples have a creepy talent to pop up right before the important event, such as prom, job interview, important public appearance, or even a date. This is no random incidence: as you will learn in the next chapter, acne has a great deal to do with stress as well as with nutrition. By using stress relieving techniques along with our Acne Detox you can stop pimples from ruining your big day, no matter what it is.

Acne Detox is a gentle and effective way to cleanse your skin from inside out. Whenever you have an important event simply set aside three days that will transform your skin. You can also try this detox before starting the Clear Acne Diet.

3 Day Acne Detox: every day for three days

On rising:
½ liter spring/mineral/purified water with 1 tsp of apple cider vinegar

Breakfast:
1 glass Skin Cleansing Drink
1 oz steel-cut oats cooked with water
1 cup green tea

Lunch
1 glass Skin Cleansing Drink
Any green salad with chicken and turkey from Clear Acne Diet
1 cup green tea
1 glass water

Mid-afternoon snack
1 cup watermelon chunks
1 glass water

Dinner (before 7 PM)
1 glass water with honey
Any green salad with chicken, turkey or tofu from Clear Acne Diet
Chamomile and peppermint herbal tea

Before bedtime
1 sliced apple with honey
1 glass Skin Cleansing Drink

Skin Cleansing Drink recipe: (never been published before)
1 lemon
1 glasses of orange juice or 1 orange
1 liter of mineral/spring/purified water
1 tbsp of maple syrup
½ inch of fresh ginger
2 tbsp virgin olive oil
1 clove of garlic, chopped
¼ tsp of cayenne pepper
¼ tsp ground cloves
¼ tsp parsley, chopped

Peel the lemon and the orange and cut them into chunks. Place all ingredients into the blender. Blend for 20 to 40 seconds. When everything is completely blended, strain the juice. It should be thick, so you may dilute it with mineral, spring or purified water. Drink a large glass of the cleanser drink every morning and every night before sleep. Store the remaining Skin Cleansing Drink in a jug in a refrigerator. You can add ice if desired.

Please note: Skin Cleansing Drink is not compatible with milk of any kind. It is rather thick, nourishing and loaded with vitamins, but it is not a meal replacement. However, you might feel quite full after a glass of Skin Cleansing Drink. In general, you will most benefit from a detox if you eat twice less than you usually do during these three days.

As with all recipes, we tried and tested this drink on ourselves as well as on audience members of our seminars. The Skin Cleansing Drink tastes like a thick orange juice with a bit of spice. The drink is amazingly easy to prepare (5-6 minutes total, including peeling and chopping) and the ingredients are quite affordable, too.

Results of Acne Detox may vary: while some people will experience greater energy and overall complexion improvement right from the start, other may feel less energetic, especially in the afternoon, while their body adjusts to the toxin elimination. However, don't be tempted to abandon the detox. To stay active, drink more green tea with honey which provides you with complex carbohydrates and energy, and add more fruits to your diet. If you truly stick to the plan, you will achieve most noticeable improvement in your skin's clarity.

Some people report that their skin blemishes get worse for the first two days. Be patient, as your skin will calm down eventually as your body gradually cleanses itself. And together with increased energy you will soon forget about cravings for fats and sugar. Please note that this detox is not intended for use during pregnancy or breast-feeding, and it's not suitable for children under 12.

Eating regularly is crucial for the success of your detox. Eat your breakfast early, not later than one hour after you get up, and allow for three hours between your next meals. If you feel hungry, take a sip of your Acne Detox Drink, eat a fruit, drink more water (ideally 1 glass every hour), green tea or diluted fruit juices to stay alert and positively minded.

CLEAR SKIN THROUGH RELAXATION

Stress is closely linked to acne. When we are stressed out, no matter by which factors, be it a traffic jam, fight with a co-worker, or an approaching deadline, our body reacts to the stress with an age-old mechanism: releasing a portion of cortisol hormones. These hormones were very helpful in primitive times when a man had to survive life-threatening situations on a daily basis, being attacked by vicious animals and suffering from the lack of food in colder months.

There are two kinds of stress we encounter on a daily basis. A positive stress accompanies us during the most exciting moments of our live: the first kiss, the wedding, the successful exam, the long-awaited promotion. Negative stress is more common. It results from boredom, insecurity, hopelessness, fear, anger, and anxiety. Negative stress ruins your health. It can result in heart diseases, digestive problems, obesity, and many skin conditions including acne. Why does it happen?

When we encounter a stress factor, our body starts working in high gear. Eye pupils dilate, so that we can see the enemy better; ears move, so the hearing is improved; breathing becomes faster. When reacting to stress, our body becomes a little power plant: it pumps up adrenaline, raises blood sugar and blood pressure, increases muscle tension and speeds up metabolism rates. That's why we loose weight when we suffer from a loss or deal with a troubled divorce, for example. During a well-documented study doctors found that student patients with acne may experience worsening of their acne during examinations. What's more, the more stress they experienced, the worse their acne became[63].

This response to stress is vital for surviving, and we all have a survivor gene that triggers the stress reaction even when we no longer hunt (or being hunted by) prehistoric tigers. But when our ancestor could release this extra energy by killing a beast or running away from danger, we don't have this luxury today. Rarely do we react to stress by doing something physical, like smashing the wall—or someone's face. More often, we suffer from stress in silence, while our body works the same powerful way as it did million years ago, producing stress-related stimulants.

During the stress the body produces the increased levels of stress substances, corticosteroids, catecholamine, and certain opiates, which suppress the immune system in general[38]. This is why stress aggravates all the inflammatory processes in your body, be it asthma, flu or acne. Stress lowers the body's resistance to bacteria and viruses and suspends tissue repair and inhibits the immune system, making us more susceptible to various viral diseases. Making your hormones go awry, stress suppresses the reproductive system which results in impotency in men and menstrual disorders in women.

There is a lot of clinical evidence suggesting that emotional stress can influence the course of acne. Doctors today believe that anxiety and even depression may not only be a result of acne but can itself makes acne worse. Stress-induced hormone cortisol released by our bodies in anxious and stressful situations stimulate the adrenal gland so it releases too much male hormone, which in turn stimulates the over-production of oil by sebum glands. But androgens are not the only stimulators of the sebaceous gland. Doctors today believe that stress-activated neuromediators, or cell surface receptors, can also intensify sebum production through complex molecular mechanism aiming sebum glands specifically. The newest finding proves that stress itself can cause acne.

In addition, people in stressful situations tend to idly pick at their pimples. But this can be harmful, increasing the possibility of infection and in the long run making the acne spot heal longer and more likely to result in scarring. Stress worsens acne marks by slowing down the healing process of the blemishes you already have. It has been estimated that in people who are under a lot of stress wounds heal 40% slower than in calm and relaxed people.

While chronic stress is disastrous to health, some stress can be in fact beneficial. A healthy dose of fear helps us make that one extra step in meeting the deadline, succeeding in the exam or completing that brilliant presentation. Doctors found that acute psychological stressors and physical exercise have been shown to rapidly enhance immune response. A little bit of positive stress is good, it helps you achieve, compete and win. Wedding is a great example of a positive stress! But when you are unhappy, easily irritated, depressed, sleepless, and have acne, then it's time to do something.

You can never completely avoid stress, but you can reduce it. I do not suggest that you quit your high-impact job, or cancel your date, or that you should start taking stress-relieving prescription drugs if you want to get rid of acne. Luckily, there are less extreme measures to reduce stress and calm down your nerves. Regular exercise helps to release tensions instead of letting them build up inside. Proper vitamin intake from a balanced diet or vitamin supplements is also important for maintaining the body's resistance to stress. Research has shown that vitamins A, B, C, and E and the minerals zinc and selenium can help keep the body's defenses strong. It's important to get enough sleep and be well rested. Spending only ten minutes a day practicing relaxation techniques will help you stay focused and calm when facing even the most complicated life situations.

HORMONES AND ACNE

Hormones are chemical messengers that transmit information from your brain to your body organs. Hormones help us stay active, burn carbohydrates and proteins, develop muscle tone, cope with stress and reproduce. There are two types of hormones that are solely responsible for acne: stress hormones and androgens, or sex hormones. We already know that stress is disastrous for your skin and overall well-being. Now let's talk about sex.

There are many hormones that have a direct impact on our skin: androgens such as dihydrotestosterone (DHT) and testosterone, the adrenal precursor dehydroepiandrosterone sulfate (DHEAS), estrogens such as estradiol, and other hormones, including growth hormone and insulin-like growth factors (IGFs), may be important in acne[39]. Sex hormone levels are produced in high quantities by adrenal glands, testis (in men) and ovaries (in women) during puberty and cause the sebaceous glands to enlarge and increase production of sebum. This process doesn't end after prom. When the oil-producing glands are over-stimulated by androgens, for example around the time of monthly periods, women of all ages are especially prone to have acne flare-ups. According to a study, most (63%) women showed a 25% premenstrual increase in the number of inflammatory acne lesions[40]. Premenstrual flares may be more common in older women: another robust study has shown that women older than 33 years had a higher rate of premenstrual acne break-outs compared to women aged 20 to 33 years[41].

Often acne signals about some endocrine hormone-related diseases. Acne is a common symptom of polycystic ovary syndrome (PCOS). During this syndrome multiple tiny cysts form in ovaries, preventing them from functioning normally. Other symptoms of PSOS include irregular periods, excess weight, thinning hair, mood swings, migraine, and more. As a result of hormonal imbalance, ovaries do not produce as much of female hormone estrogen as needed to counterbalance the male hormone testosterone. The excess of testosterone results in increased oiliness of the skin (men's skin is naturally more oily and thick), increased body hair growth, menstrual irregularities (too heavy or less frequent), obesity or anorexia, and acne.

To oppose the effects of androgens on the skin doctors often prescribe hormonal therapy. Hormones may be used in acne even if there are no endocrine abnormalities. While severe acne requires antiandrogens such as cyproterone acetate or aldactone, mild or moderate acne benefits from hormonal contraceptives[42]. In case of polycystic ovarian syndrome many doctors today recommend exercise and diet to lose weight because excess weight is often associated with this disorder. It is important for dermatologists to work closely with gynecologists so that women with polycystic ovary syndrome don't face the risks of cardiovascular disease, insulin-resistant diabetes, and infertility.

BEWARE OF ACNE-RELATED DEPRESSION

Acne has a huge impact on your emotions, and vice versa. Lowered self-esteem, ruined relationships, anxiety, unemployment, self-consciousness, embarrassment, frustration and negative body image—acne contributes to all the above. The recent study revealed a shocking truth: among fifty acne patients nineteen of them (38 per cent) were suffering from depression, most of them women. Social anxiety was also prevalent in acne patients (34 per cent). Most dangerously, among nineteen depressed patients four of them (whopping 21 per cent!) admitted having suicidal thoughts[43].

Acne has a huge impact on well-being. People with acne may tend to underestimate themselves, loosing confidence and positive outlook. They often see themselves as ugly and undesirable, which leads to inadequate social behavior. Some acne sufferers grow their hair long to cover the face. Girls tend to wear heavy make-up to disguise the pimples, even though they know this sometimes aggravates the condition. Many boys affected with acne avoid sport activities because of the need to undress in changing rooms.

Acne may also result in social withdrawal. Many acne sufferers think that their acne pimples are disgusting and blame acne for communication and personal problems which leads to further alienation. This is why acne sufferers even stop dating for the fear of rejection. They avoid public appearances and even change careers to stay away from people. They are hardly to blame: acne pimples, especially when they affect the face, provoke pitiless jokes from other teenagers.

Acne affects career and education, too. Some acne sufferers refuse to go school which may result in poor academic performance and possibly future unemployment. Adults with acne take sick days from work, risking their jobs. Acne may reduce career choices, ruling out occupations such as modeling, acting, public relations that depend upon personal appearance. Acne sufferers are less successful in job applications for two reasons: first, they lack confidence; second, potential employers have generally negative reaction to their unhealthy skin. More people who have acne are unemployed than people who do not have acne are[44].

But the biggest harm acne makes to the person's soul. Acne sufferers tend to blame themselves for their skin disorders, and their anger turns two directions: inwards, when they blame and even punish themselves for those pimples; and outwards, when the rage explodes hurting family members, friends, colleagues and even strangers. Recent studies show that people with acne have more active suicidal thoughts as a result of depression.

Depression and suicidal thoughts are strikingly common among acne sufferers, note the researchers[45]. Dangerous signs of depression can include persistent negativity or increased moodiness and irritability, loss or increase of appetite, trouble sleeping or sleeping too much, lack of energy, avoiding friends, social isolation, and negative thoughts that range from feeling helpless and lonely to thoughts of worthlessness, self-harm or suicide. Rarely, depression can be associated with acne treatment, particularly isotretinoin. Regardless of the cause, depression must be recognized and managed early. If you think you may be depressed, contact your dermatologist or family doctor urgently for advice.

TAKE YOUR SKIN TO THE SHRINK

Dermatologists have long suspected that acne and skin problems like rosacea, hives and psoriasis are linked to the stress. And they have not been ignoring this knowledge. Many dermatologists today ask about a patient's current state of emotional affairs when dealing with such skin problems as acne, rosacea, and eczema. There is even a new field of medicine developing, a psychodermatology. Even though it's not official, this approach of linking traditional dermatology and emotional heath has proven to be effective. "Skin-emotion specialist" may be a psychiatrist, psychologist, social worker, biofeedback therapist, or other mental health or behavioral specialist[46].

Psychocutaneous medicine or the medicine that treats skin problems addressing mental issues first, is being incorporated into the mainstream medical practice today. Many people, who are frequently not satisfied with traditional medical therapies, opt for psychocutaneous intervention which may result in less flushing, less anxiety, less anger, less social embarrassment and withdrawal, and improved sleep. This technique may also bring result in improved well-being, increased sense of control, and enhanced acceptance of your appearance affected by the skin disease.

How does it work? To establish a connection between skin disorder and emotional disarray, doctors act pretty much like a psychotherapists, using psychotherapeutic stress-and-anxiety-management techniques such as hypnosis, progressive muscle relaxation, guided imagery, yoga, Tai Chi or biofeedback.

When suffering from skin disorder many people try medical solution first. But sometimes medicine, be it prescription or over the counter, doesn't provide much relief. If you suspect you might have some deep-rooted emotional issues that keep your acne treatment of choice from effectively clearing your skin, you may want to explore relaxation techniques.

CLEAR SKIN WITH STRESS RELIEF

If you got used to the idea that acne treatment must involve antibiotics and harsh cleansers in order to be effective, you are wrong. The very idea of Acne Detox instead of pimple lotion seems weird enough. But in fact, a human body has an incredible ability to change itself using help from inside and outside. Just like a member of Mutant X clan, you can change your physical state by taking some Valium or drowning a bottle of vodka. You can beat cold by popping vitamin C pills. You can lose several pounds on juice fasting. By entering a state of self-induced trance athletes can run exhausting marathons and set world records with little-known secrets of self-hypnosis. Similarly, stress-relieving exercise and simple techniques that address the subconscious mind will help you rid of negative emotional baggage that is extremely dangerous to your health in general and skin in particular.

Deep Breathing Exercises

Breathing is the only bodily function that we can consciously control. When we are stressed, we breathe in rapid, shallow strokes. When we are asleep or relaxed on the beach we inhale and exhale the air slowly and effortlessly, allowing greater quantities of air enter the lungs and more oxygen traveling to various organs—including the skin. That is why deep controlled breathing is crucial to stress relief and acne treatment. Deep breathing helps focus the mind, balance the emotions, and get more oxygen into the blood stream. Breathing exercises don't require any equipment to practice so you can do them in the office, at home or even during a lunch break.

For the beginning try to perform the following breathing exercises in a warm quiet place, wearing comfortable unrestricted clothes while sitting or lying in a comfortable position. Lay down on your back, with shoulders firmly on the floor. Place your hands right on the belly button stretching the fingers out. Now, take a deep breath through your nostrils and feel how your abdomen expands and stomach area protrudes. Make sure your chest doesn't rise and shoulders remain pressed to the floor. Breathe out through your mouth and try to push out all the air from your lungs.

Take ten deep breathes and relax breathing normally. Don't rush yourself, or you will end up with dizziness and hyperventilation. When you get used to breathing right, you can start deep breathing in the fresh air, in the park or at the balcony. Another exercise would be imagining the fresh air flowing through your body, entering the brain and dissolving your worries. Enjoy the fresh air as it melts down your stress, penetrates your skin, and evaporates away through lungs and pores as you exhale. Isn't it wonderful?

When I started regular breathing exercises, my face regained healthy pinkish glow. Very calming and soothing, breathing exercises never fail to instantly unwind me, no matter when and where. In stressful situations breathing exercises help me keep clear thinking and allow me stay in control of my emotions. I practice deep breathing every morning walking my dog in the park, during the lunch break enjoying the weather, and I never miss the change to have a powerful deep breathing session during a vacation on the seaside, when salty flavorful air power-cleanses my lungs.

Meditation

Meditation helps improve concentration, calms the mind, and balances the nervous system. There are many meditation techniques, and all of them are really simple. The breathing exercise can be practiced during the meditation.

Meditation can be enjoyed by anyone. You don't have to be a yogi, or an adept of mystical teachings, or even a deeply religious person. Meditation in one or another form has been practiced by people of all religions for centuries.

To meditate, find a quiet place in your home. Close your eyes and perform a breathing exercise for ten minutes. Concentrate on the breath—make sure your lungs are completely empty before inhaling again. Listen to the sounds closest to you—your own breath, your heart rate or maybe a distant noise of traffic or sounds of a wind. Gradually listen to the sounds that are further away—the trees outside, the airplanes, or distant car honks. Imagine you can hear sounds that are even further away—dogs barking a mile away, the ocean hundreds of miles away. Let yourself float away trying to catch those distant sounds. Breathe deeply and slowly and keep your body absolutely relaxed.

There's another type of meditation which is more helpful for those who find it hard to concentrate. Start with performing both breathing techniques. Close your eyes and concentrate on one single word. It could be your name, a pleasant yet meaningless sound, or something common in meditation such as "ohm." Think of the sound of the word and shapes of the letters. Don't let your mind wander—concentrate on one single word and constantly return to it.

With practice, you will no longer need to think of associated words and will be able to concentrate on the single word for fifteen minutes or even more.

If you find it hard to concentrate on a word, concentrate on a visual image, such as imaginary peaceful sunset on a beach or a flame of a candle. Try to remember all the colors, smells, sounds and even tiny details. With candle, lit a candle, plain or aromatherapeutic, and look at the flame. Concentrate on its shape, movement, scents and tiny crackling sounds. Soon you will feel warm and light feeling inside. Enjoy it. You are meditating and your worries and acne are melting away!

I particularly like the Dalai Lama meditation technique. Close your eyes and imagine yourself as people see you—as if you look in the mirror. Then try imagining empty bulletin board in front of you. Next, envision yourself angry and place this picture to the left side of your mental bulletin board. Then picture yourself calm and peaceful, and place this picture to the right side of your mental bulletin board. Next, picture yourself, say, drunk. Place this disturbing image to the left side. Then, picture yourself sober and energetic. Place this image to the right side. See yourself fat and unattractive and place this sad image to the left side. Then, imagine yourself slim and sexy, and put this picture to the right. Follow this with any negative and positive images of yourself: impatient—to the left, patient and understanding—to the right. Gloomy—to the left, happy—to the right. Sad and depressed—to the left, smiling and energetic—to the right. Then look at all those sad, ugly, stupid pictures on the left. Do you hate them? Then look at happy, glowing, smiling you on the right. This is the person you want to be. Soon your subconscious will be disgusted with the negative image of yours, and slowly, without even realizing it, you will step by step move towards the happy positive imagery on the right side of your mental bulletin board.

This type of meditation is using the power of subconscious that reprograms your inner world. Many stresses are results of negative messages sent by subconscious. If you learn to control and employ your subconscious you can become relaxed and much healthier.

Clear Skin Affirmations

Subconscious is a powerful force and gaining control over your subconscious can make wonders to your well-being and looks. Most problems caused by stress are result of subconscious working against you. Subconscious can adopt and make real virtually any suggestion repeated over a time especially under favorable conditions, for example, when you are half-asleep.

Just like a hypnotist brings us into a state of trance and makes us follow his commands, we can also hypnotize ourselves, and we do it on a daily basis. Tell yourself that you feel tired for ten times in a row, and you will indeed feel sleepy and weak. Tell yourself you will never ever scratch your back, and you will feel such a powerful urge to scratch you won't be able to stand it. This has nothing to do with willpower. This is your imagination working. The more you tell yourself you are *not* going to scratch your back, the more you will long for that one simple pleasure. However, you can manipulate the way you think and feel just as easily, pushing positive ideas into your subconscious. This is simple, but requires repetition and persistence.

Most of acne sufferers want to feel like a beautiful self-confident well-accepted people while the subconscious makes them believe we are continuously been ignored, given a cold shoulder and generally disliked. And since the cold truth (a new juicy zit or an array of blackheads) stares at us from any mirror, there's no use teaching yourself "I am the most beautiful person on earth." Subconscious won't buy that. Instead, tell yourself "My blemishes are healing faster" or "My skin is getting clearer every minute." Construct your affirmations as simple positive present time sentences, and they will work wonders for you.

When trying to influence your subconscious avoid complex sentences and sub-clauses. Instead, repeat one simple affirmation over and over again. Just like a hyperactive actor in TV infomercials or a guru from self-help audio tape, repeat same thing at least 10 times literally pushing the right ideas inside your subconscious. In order to use Clear Skin Affirmations in the most effective way you should work them out ahead of time, word them properly, and memorize.

This is how your clear skin affirmation may look like: **"I am relaxing and feeling peaceful and calm. My complexion is healing faster. My skin is becoming clear and radiant. More and more, I feel my face getting clear. I radiate beauty and self-confidence to all people I meet."**

The best time to practice Clear Skin Affirmations is when you put yourself in a state of self-hypnosis. Here's a self-hypnosis technique adapted from a Betty Erickson technique. I found it very easy to follow.

This self-hypnosis technique offers a pre-hypnotic suggestion. In other words, you tell yourself what you want to accomplish before you go into the self-induced trance.

1. Get comfortable. Sit or lay down on the floor. Practice deep breathing for three minutes.

2. Now tell yourself how exactly you will act when you have reached the state of trance. Tell yourself several times, **"I am going into a trance to repeat my affirmations. During this self-hypnosis session I will repeat my affirmations twenty times helping my skin heal naturally and easily."** You can also tell yourself that your eyes will close the moment you have reached the moment of trance. This will work as a proof that your mind is ready to accept your affirmations.

3. Now, tell yourself how you want to feel when you complete the process and how long you wish to be in a trance, **"In twenty minutes, I'm going to wake up, feeling rested and calm."**

4. Focus your eyes on something bright and pleasant-looking. It may be a flower in a vase or a spot of light on the wall.

5. Now, keeping your eyes focused on the bright spot, notice three things (one at a time) that you see. Tell yourself what you see. Now notice, one by one, three things that you hear. Next, notice three sensations. Go slowly from one to the next. You can use sensations that normally are outside of your awareness, such as the temperature of your hands, the feeling of the floor under your feet, the pressure of your waistband, and so on.

6. Now, repeat the process but note only two things you see, hear and feel. Next, just one sound and two feelings. Now see one thing and feel one thing only.

7. Now you will probably notice that your eyes have closed on their own accord. Now you have opened up your subconscious mind at least a little bit and

are ready to apply suggestions. Repeat the affirmations you know by heart. Your subconscious will do the rest.

Alternatively, you may record your affirmations on a tape recorder. In this case, you may tell yourself before starting the self-hypnosis session that "I will turn on tape recorder." This way, you will listen to your affirmations without having to memorize them. However, I would suggest that you make an effort and memorize those five short sentences.

8. When you are done reciting your affirmations, you can terminate your session. Resist the urge to just open your eyes and get up. You should make a clear termination to your self-hypnosis session so that it doesn't affect your clear consciousness. To end the session, think to yourself that you are going to be fully awake after you count up to, say, three. Tell yourself, **"One, I'm beginning wake up. Two, I'm becoming more awake. Three, I'm completely awake."**

Don't nap immediately after self-hypnosis session, or your mind will link sleeping with self-hypnosis practice. It's a good idea to set up a schedule of practice, allowing yourself anywhere between 10 and 30 minutes, depending on how busy you are and how much time you have to spend at it.

Practice self-hypnosis and Clear Skin Affirmations during the least busy part of your day, when you are least likely to be disturbed by phone calls or family members. Assign yourself at least 30 minutes for each session. Affirmations and self-hypnosis can do wonders to your well-being and looks if you practice this technique regularly and enthusiastically.

Clear Skin Face Massage

Self-massage is a proven way to relieve stress, boost blood circulation, improve your complexion, and leave your face looking fresher. You don't have to be a certified masseuse to practice self-massage: these simple movements are easy to learn and apply.

Before you begin, get some face massage oil so you don't pull your skin. The ideal face massage oils for acne-prone skin include evening primrose, calendula kernel, and jojoba oils. Grape seed oil is especially good for people with nut allergies. If you don't like the feeling of oil on your skin, you can wash your face after the massage. Spread a few drops of oil between your palms and rub your hands vigorously to warm up the oil.

1. Start with deep breathing and relaxation. To block out the sounds of the outside world, turn on some soothing music. Close your eyes.

2. Cover your eyes with your hands, with heels of your palms just under your cheekbones. Apply a light pressure and hold this position for 15 seconds. Then slowly move your palms to the sides of your face, stretching (but not pulling!) your skin as you move. Repeat this exercise 5 times.

3. Tilt your head to one side and place your relaxed fingers on the side of your neck. Using your fingers stroke from the chin to the collarbone, one hand following the other. Gently move the skin in a downwards direction. When you reach the shoulder, use a gentle movement around the front of your neck in towards the top of your breastbone, where the collarbones meet. This exercise boosts the lymph drainage from your face. Repeat 10 times on each side of your neck.

4. Pinch your jaw line using your thumbs and index fingers. Start under your chin and work out toward your ears. Make sure you don't stretch the skin. Repeat 3 pinching sessions at each side of your face.

5. Stimulate the skin by using the back of your hands and loosely rolling your fingers up the cheek. Be gentle if you have pimples. Repeat 5 times at each side of your face.

6. Now find an acupressure point approximately 1 cm (1/2 inch) between your nostril and cheekbones. Apply a light pressure for 15 seconds. Then slowly stroke your fingers up the nose reaching the eyebrow bone and glide your fingers to the temple area. Repeat 10 times.

7. Stroke in a circle around your eyes with your ring fingers. Stroke firmly and evenly from the bridge of your nose out over your eyebrows, press on your temples, and then glide gently under your eyes, barely touching the skin. This exercise helps diminish under-eye circles. Repeat 6 times at each eye.

8. Gently drag your fingers across forehead from the bridge of your nose to your hairline with one hand following the other. Repeat 5 times.

9. Then spread your fingers across your temple area, forming a "claw", then apply a light pressure and draw them over the forehead, into the hairline and up to the crown of the head. Slowly lift and repeat the action. This time, there would be almost no oil left on your hands, so you won't make your hair greasy. Repeat 10 times.

10. Finish the self-massaging session by cupping your eyes with palms of your hands. Put the heel of your hands into your eye sockets and hold your hands there for a few seconds without any pressure at all. Enjoy the darkness but avoid pressing so hard so that you start seeing white dots. Hold the position for 10 seconds, and then slowly glide your hands away. You can rest, with your eyes closed, for as long as you feel comfortable.

Regular practice of relaxation methods can help prevent stress before it happens. Learning to relax more will greatly help to reduce stress-related acne. Every day take time to read a book, listen to music, have a bath, go for a walk, enjoy your hobby, whatever it takes for you to unwind and de-stress. If you get used to relax, you'll find yourself being able to achieve more, because you will be more rested and energized.

CLEAN SKINCARE FOR HEALTHY SKIN

Our life is overloaded with chemicals. We eat chemically enhanced food, we drink water of questionable quality, and we inhale pollutants every minute. According to Environmental Protection Agency, indoor air is two to five times more polluted than the air outside. Building materials, furnishings, carpet, household cleaning products, and chemical air refreshers all add up to already dangerous mix of radon, pesticides, and outdoor air pollution[47].

As if it weren't enough, every woman is exposed to a whopping amount of chemicals lurking in her skincare and makeup products. Statistics say that an average North American woman owns about five hundred dollars' worth of cosmetic products. That's a lot! After a quick count of chemical ingredients containing in the typical cleanser, toner, moisturizer, eye cream, facial scrub, body wash, body lotion, and sunscreen, I came up with more than two hundred different chemicals that an average woman applies to her skin daily! Unfortunately, most skincare products we use today are formulated with synthetic and sometimes toxic ingredients. Dangerous and mostly unstudied for safety, they can create new toxic compounds when they interact with each other.

Out skin can easily absorb chemicals, no matter good or bad. According to the recent research more than 60 per cent of topically applied chemicals are absorbed by skin and spread all over the body with the bloodstream[48]. Doctors use this ability to deliver medications transdermally, for example, in nicotine and contraceptive patches. And since the skin is the largest organ in our body and it soaks up toxic chemical contaminants in much larger amounts than intestines or lungs[49].

Toxic chemicals that penetrate the skin may provoke irritation and inflammation of the skin especially when they are intensively rubbed into skin (scrubs, cleansers) or left on skin for a long time (moisturizers, toners). And while ecological matters are often beyond our control, we can reduce the exposure to harmful chemicals by carefully choosing products we wash, scrub, tone, moisturize and rejuvenate our skin.

Most skin care products on the market today contain hundreds of synthetic additives that are in most cases not proven safe to use. There are over 100,000 various chemicals in use all over the world, and while there are certain regulations when it comes to industrial-strength toxic chemicals, no one is able to calculate the risks of using the same toxic chemicals in small doses over many years. No one can tell which impact on health a daily use of SPF50 sunblock may have in ten years from now—apart from pale skin—simply because these sunblocks have been introduced not so long ago. Beauty products are most often tested on mice or rabbits whose lifespan is rather limited compared to the one of a man. Human studies conducted by manufacturers often focus on overall appeal such as pleasant smell, a light texture or short-term results, such as "instant lifting effect."

Unfortunately, many cosmetic manufacturers use not only toxic, but potentially carcinogenic ingredients that increase our risk of having a cancer at some point in our lives. As if breathing polluted air and eating chemicals was not enough! When you apply a skincare product that contains these ingredients, all these potentially cancer-causing poisonous chemicals are absorbed by the skin and carried with blood all over the body. The poisonous chemical can also interact with other chemicals in our bodies. Sometimes these chemical reactions produce substances that promote cells to evolve in a wrong way resulting in cancer.

Toxic ingredients may lead to many other serious diseases. including allergies, fertility problems, diabetes and Alzheimer's disease. In best-case scenario, they may worsen existing acne or may cause an allergic reaction that resembles acne. That's why we sometimes "break out" after using a new cream or a cleanser.

Here's how certain chemicals affect your acne:

- Toxic chemical ingredients disrupt hormonal balance. Hormonal glands activated by chemicals send frequent signals to all bodily systems, including sebum glands, which results in sebum overproduction and increased shedding of pore lining which both contribute to acne.

- Chemicals such as silicones clog pores blocking the excretion of sebum which triggers the acne reaction.

- Chemicals such as petrolatum (mineral oil) coat the skin with artificial grease which doesn't allow skin function normally expelling toxins and moisturizing itself using its own sebum.

- Some chemicals enhance the penetration of the skin product which exposes the body to even greater amount of toxic substances. In addition, they may irritate the skin starting the micro-inflammation inside the pore or increasing the existing inflammation.

No wonder that skin conditions such as eczema, allergic dermatitis and acne are on the rise. Most often, acne today is aggravated not by diet or stress, but by specific ingredients in our skincare and body care products. We need to identify and avoid them in order to rebalance our skin just like we rebalanced our emotions and diet earlier.

Below is a list of chemical ingredients commonly found in skincare and makeup. You will often find these chemicals both in drugstore products that cost $3 and in high-end creams and serums that carry $100+ price tag.

20 DANGEROUS SKINCARE INGREDIENTS TO AVOID

The amount of toxins in our environment has reached a level where the FDA now has designated "permissible" levels of harmful chemicals in food and cosmetics. However, you will not find any warnings on the cosmetic label. Neither will you find worst of these chemicals in ingredient lists. They are usually listed in small print and typed in all caps so that you will have trouble deciphering the label. Sometimes these deadly chemical ingredients are hiding under abbreviations or safe-sounding and even organic names.

DIOXIN

Found in PEG, Polyethylene, Polyethylene Glycol, Polyoxyethylene, Oxynol, Nonoxynol, Polysorbate 60, Polysorbate 80

Dioxins are a group of persistent, very toxic chemicals that form during production of pharmaceuticals, cosmetics, detergents, plastic packaging and some dyes. The worst thing about dioxin is that it bioaccumulates in the body. This means that the body accumulates any dioxin to which you are exposed, so even small amounts of dioxins may accumulate to dangerous levels over years. Dioxin components were first shown to cause liver cancer in lab animals in studies of National Cancer Institute in 1970s.

Dioxin is a powerful hormone disruptor that mimics estrogen hormones in the body. Dioxin exposure can damage the immune system and can lead to increased cancer risks, as well as infertility, birth defects, impaired child development, diabetes, and thyroid changes. Because hormones and immune system are constantly off balance, acne occurs.

FDA admits that "many foaming cleansers and cosmetic emulsifiers identifiable by the prefix, word or syllable "PEG," "Polyethylene," "Polyethylene glycol," "Polyoxyethylene," "-eth-," or "-oxynol," may be contaminated with 1.4-dioxane.[10] Such ingredients are often found in shampoos and bubble baths listed as PEG, polyethylene, polyethylene glycol, polyoxyethylene, oxynol, nonoxynol, polysorbate 60 and polysorbate 80. Chemical industry uses higher levels of ethylene oxide to decrease the irritancy factor in baby shampoos.

NITROSAMINES

Compounds found on majority of cosmetic labels

Nitrosamines are not present in cosmetic products, but they are formed by a chemical reaction during application or when the product sits on store shelf. Ingredients that form nitrosamines include diethanolamine (DEA), triethanolamine (TEA), hydrolyzed animal protein, and padimate-O (octyl dimethyl PABA). Shampooing the hair with a product contaminated with nitrosamine can lead to its absorption into the body at levels much higher than eating nitrite-contaminated foods.

More than 100,000 tons of diethanolamine (DEA) are sold in the United States each year. It is used as a wetting or thickening agent in not only shampoos but also such products as hand soaps, hairsprays and sunscreens. My recent browse through Lancome counter shows that triethanolamine is present in every product, from toner to eye cream!

Other nitrosamine-forming compounds include lauramide siethanolamine, coco diethanolamide, coconut oil amide of diethanolamine, lauramide DEA, lauric diethanolamide, lauroyl diethanolamide, and lauryl diethanolamide.

Most nitrosamines have been shown to penetrate the skin when applied even in smallest amounts. They are potent carcinogens—substances that promote cancerous tumor growth. Recent studies show that diethanolamine (DEA), commonly found in shampoos and conditioners, slowed down the brain formation in fetuses of pregnant mice. At this point it is a caution. The dose of DEA a person might get from shampooing is at least 10 times lower than the dose found to interfere with brain development in the study. However, no one has ever measured the dose of DEA after ten shampoos or after a year of daily shampooing with DEA-rich shampoo. This is why doctors recommend expectant mothers to look at product labels and try to limit exposure to DEA until science knows more.

Addition of antioxidants, such as vitamin C and tocopherol (vitamin E), may slow, but will not prevent, the formation of nitrosamines. However, in order to avoid jeopardizing your health you may wish to avoid skincare products containing ethanolamines in any form.

POLYETHYLENE GLYCOLS

Found on majority of cosmetic labels

These toxic petroleum-based surfactants are commonly used in cosmetics. Propylene glycol is used in moisturizers and cleansers as a humectant, an ingredient that draws moisture to skin. Most often you can identify them by letters "PEG" followed by a number.

Propylene glycol is a powerful penetration enhancer which allows chemicals be absorbed better by the skin. The EPA considers propylene glycol so toxic that it requires workers to wear protective gloves, clothing and goggles when they work with this substance. Because propylene glycol penetrates the skin so quickly, the EPA warns against skin contact to prevent consequences such as brain, liver, and kidney abnormalities. But there isn't even a warning label on products such as stick deodorants, where the **concentration is greater than in most industrial applications.** There is a higher dose of ethylene glycols in children shampoos and baby washes so they become less irritating to baby's whisper-thin skin.

SODIUM LAUREL SULFATE

Found in facial cleansers, shampoos, bath foams

This is a harsh foaming agent is the major skin offender. It is derived from petroleum which sometimes is masked with phrase "comes from coconuts." However, sodium laurel sulphate in fact is composed with four known carcinogens: formaldehyde, dioxane, ethylene oxide, and acetaldehyde. No wonder it causes eye irritation, skin rashes and allergic reactions, in addition to being potentially carcinogenic.

PETROLATUM/LIQUID PARAFFIN/MINERAL OIL

Found in facial and body moisturizers, serums, masks, sunblocks

All these familiar names belong to petroleum family of chemicals. "Petroleum family is like any family," says Leanne McCliskie of Dermalogica, "There are great members and there are some completely awful ones." While silicones tend to behave better on skin, petrolatum and liquid paraffin are particularly nasty.

These petroleum derivatives are used for their emollient properties in moisturizers.

Petrolatum is very popular due to its unbelievable low price. You can find mineral oil (a posh synonym of petrolatum) both in drugstore facial lotions, baby oil and even Crème de la Mer! Basically, petrolatum is restricted in EU cosmetics. This chemical forms a film on the skin surface that can interfere with the body's own natural moisturizing mechanism. It results in dryness and increased skin cell shedding which promotes acne and other disorders. Petrolatum also slows down skin function and cell development, resulting in premature aging. Petrolatum is a major skin abuser, so stay away from it!

FORMALDEHYDE

Found in mascara, nail polish

Formaldehyde is considered a carcinogen, according to both EPA and the National Toxicology. In liquid state formaldehyde can be found in polyquaternium-15, DMDM Hydantoin, and Diazolidinyl Urea. These ingredients can be absorbed through skin and nail bed. You can also inhale formaldehyde when someone else does your manicure or pedicure.

PARABENS

Found in nearly all cosmetic products

Parabens are used as preservatives because they can prohibit microbial growth and extend shelf life of products. Studies have shown that parabens are easily absorbed by the body through the skin. They have estrogenic properties and are known to be toxic. Parabens are often touted as "food-grade preservatives" which doesn't make them any safer or less potent. Parabens are proven endocrine disruptors raising concern for impaired fertility or development. Parabens are widely banned in European cosmetics, and there is a chance they will be banned in North America as well, because the recent studies found parabens concentrated in breast cancer tumors.

DIAZOLIDINYL/IMIDAZOLIDINYL UREA

Found in shampoos, facial cleansers, moisturizers, masks and eye creams

These are most commonly used preservatives after the parabens. The American Academy of Dermatology considers them to be the primary cause of contact dermatitis in people. When diazolidinyl/imidazolidinyl urea reacts with another preservative it releases formaldehyde, which is an immune system toxicant and sensitizer that instigates immune system response that can include itching, burning, scaling, hives, and blistering of skin.

D & C RED PIGMENTS

Found in skin toners, shampoos, eye shadows, facial powders, foundations, lipsticks

These pigments are synthetic colors made from coal tar which contains heavy metal salts. They deposit toxins onto the skin, causing skin sensitivity and irritation. Animal studies have shown almost all of them to be carcinogenic. All of D & C Red dyes tested to date, the xanthenes, monoazoanilines, fluorans, and indigoids, are comedogenic. D & C Red dyes are often used in blush and are responsible for cosmetic acne in the cheekbone area. All D & C Red dyes are dangerous to some extent, but the most hazardous type of D & C pigments is D & C Red No. 9 which is a proven carcinogen. The natural red pigment, carmine, however, is non-comedogenic and works well as a substitute for D & C dyes in blushers.[50]

PHENOXYETHANOL

Found in facial cleansers, toners, moisturizers, eye creams, serums

Phenoxyethanol is a synthetic ether alcohol preservative. Recent studies show that phenoxyethanol is a reproductive or developmental toxin which is thought to possible present risks to human reproduction and development. This chemical is linked to potential for reduced fertility or reduced chance for a healthy, full-term pregnancy. Today many organic and semi-organic brands use phenoxyethanol derived from grapefruit, so if you see mostly natural ingredients on the label and phenoxyethanol among them, don't panic: plant-derived phenoxyethanol may be perfectly safe.

PABA (para-aminobenzoic acid, Padimate-O, octyl dimethyl PABA)

Found in sunscreens, facial moisturizers with SPF

Limited scientific evidence shows that in fact PABA may increase the chances of getting skin cancer because it absorbs the UV radiation rays and encourages forming of free radicals. It may may cause formation of nitrosamines which are potentially carcinogenic.

TALC

Found in foundations, powders, eye shadows, blushers, bronzers, lipsticks, baby powders

Talc, or talcum powder, is a known respiratory toxicant widely used in skin foundations and powders. Talc may contain asbestos fibers which are linked to cancer. In addition to that, scientific studies have shown that routine application of talc in the genital area of baby girls is associated with a three-to-fourfold increase in the development of ovarian cancer later in life. Do you really believe that skin in genital area is much different from skin on your face?

ISOPROPYL PALMITATE, MYRISTATE

Found in moisturizers, lip glosses, lipsticks, facial cleansers, foundations, scrubs, eye shadows, eye creams, eye makeup removers, mascara, perfumes, nail polishes

This fatty acid derived from palm oil is usually combined in skincare with synthetic alcohol. Industry tests on rabbits indicate that isopropyl palmitate can cause skin irritation, dermatitis and pore clogging which makes it acne promoting. A similar-sounding isopropyl myristate is the ester of isopropyl alcohol and myristic acid used in cosmetic to increase the absorption of the product through the skin. Isopropyl is derived from propane, a gaseous and flammable component of petroleum.

There's no need to beware of similarly sounding **myristyl myristate** which is derived from palm oil, nutmeg, or milk. Myristyl myristate is not a known carcinogen and is not known to be toxic.

TRICLOSAN

Found in acne cleansers, acne treatments, moisturizers, deodorants, body washes, toothpaste, shampoos, perfumes

This once popular antibacterial agent is now shown to be potentially contaminated with impurities linked to cancer or other significant health problems. Triclosan is also considered an immune system toxin. It can be drying to skin, causing the top layer shed dead skin cells more actively which leads to pore blockage and further spread of acne.

SILICONE

Found in moisturizers, foundations, sunscreens, eye creams, cleansers, bronzers, eye shadows, blush, lipsticks, eye makeup removers, acne treatments

Silicone emollients show up on cosmetic labels as cyclomethicone, dimethicone, trimethicone, or plant-derived silicone. They coat the skin and clog the pores, acting pretty much like a plastic wrap. Recent studies have indicated that prolonged exposure of the skin to sweat causes skin irritation and swelling of pore walls which promotes acne. Some synthetic emollients are known tumor promoters and accumulate in the liver and lymph nodes.

LANOLIN

Found in lipsticks, moisturizers, lip glosses

Lanolin is obtained from the sheep's wool, so any chemicals used on sheep will contaminate the lanolin. The majority of lanolin used in cosmetics is highly contaminated with organo-phosphate pesticides and insecticides which are known carcinogens. In addition to that lanolin is known to block pores and promote acne. Synthetic versions of lanolin have different molecular structure and they are generally harmless to acne-prone skin types.

GLYCERIN

Found in moisturizers, facial cleansers, toothpaste

Glycerin, or glycerol, is basically a sugar alcohol and is naturally present in human body as well in fats and oils. Glycerin is a popular emollient, humectant, solvent and lubricant in skincare products. Due to its ability to draw moisture from air and add it to skin glycerin can make skin drier over the long term and seal off the normal breathing of skin by clogging pores thus promoting acne.

CETEARYL ALCOHOL

Found in moisturizers, cleansers, scrubs, mascara, acne treatments

Cetearyl alcohol is not a typical alcohol we use to rub on sore spots or consume as part of alcoholic beverages. It's is a mixture of *fatty alcohols* derived from coconut or palm kernel oil, and it is used in cosmetics as an emulsion stabilizer in moisturizers and foam booster in facial cleansers. Cetearyl alcohol makes moisturizers glide luxuriously on the skin. However, it's exceptionally comedogenic and can promote acne.

CETYL ALCOHOL

Found in moisturizers, cleansers, eye creams, sunscreens, lipsticks, acne treatments, mascara, foundations

Cetyl alcohol is known under many names such as palmityl alcohol, hexadecan-1-ol hexadecanol. It's an organic fatty alcohol first derived from whale oil. It is used as an emollient, an emulsifier and thickening agent in moisturizers. Cetyl alcohol is a powerful comedogen so try to avoid it if you are prone to acne.

Studies show that these skincare ingredients **can cause problems when used frequently**, over a period of time. Avoid them whenever possible. Although a lot of these contaminant particles were initially too large to penetrate the skin, today they are able to penetrate better due to special ingredients called "penetration enhancers" such as alpha-hydroxy acids, propylene glycol, and alcohols.

When you experience an adverse reaction to a skincare product, call your local FDA office, listed in the Blue Pages of the telephone book under U.S. Department of Health and Human Services. Otherwise contact your family doctor, and if the reaction is acute and persistent, call medical emergency services.

WHY COSMETIC COMPANIES USE TOXIC CHEMICALS IN SKINCARE?

Because they can

Food and Drug Administration and Health Canada cannot possibly review all chemicals and their combinations in thousands of new beauty products, however, they have extensive lists of chemicals that cannot be used in cosmetics. Once harmful effects of chemicals are proven they are then added to these "black lists" and removed from the market. However, every year thousands of new chemicals are developed and used in cosmetics. Not all new chemicals have harmful effects but do you really want to use a product for several years only to find out later the harm that you were doing to your body?

You would be surprised to learn that in most cases the government does not require health studies or pre-market testing for cosmetics and other personal care products before they hit the $35 billion beauty market. According to the FDA's Office of Cosmetics and Colors, "cosmetics and their ingredients are not required to undergo approval before they are sold to the public." This means that manufacturers may use any ingredient or raw material, except for color additives and a few prohibited substances, to market a product without a government review or approval.

The toxicity of skincare product ingredients is tested almost exclusively by a self-policing industry safety committee, the Cosmetic Ingredient Review panel (CIR). Testing is voluntary and controlled by the manufacturers, which hardly makes the reviews unbiased. As a result, 89 percent of more than 10,500 ingredients used in personal care products have not been evaluated for safety by CIR, FDA, or any other publicly accountable institution.

Because they need to make profit

Using cheap chemicals is less expensive than trying to replace them with more expensive but less toxic natural ingredients. When I mentioned to a CEO of an "organic" skincare line that her formulation contains triethanolamine and dimethicone—both are hardly compatible with organic concept,—she was angry at first, but then admitted that she would have to spend additional half-million dollars to replace those ingredients in their whole lineup of products.

Research and development, tests, in vitro and clinical, purchase of new ingredients, adjustment of machinery, packaging redesign and perhaps new marketing campaign total into a considerable six-figure number that would be hard to justify on a price tag. On the other hand, cosmetic companies have working formulations and manufacturing processes that require little to no upkeep, maybe just a tiny tweak, such as new scent or color. Needless to say, instead of losing millions of dollars on research and reformulating products they would rather blame the sun for the dramatic rise of cancer among young women. Sun is free; chemicals aren't.

Because synthetic skincare sells better

As a matter of fact, all the deadly synthetic chemical garbage is designed to do is to make the manufactures, the CEOs and the shareholders wealthy. Triethanolamine, parabens, formaldehyde, and diazolidinyl urea increase shelf life of cosmetic products so that the fragrance and consistency of the product remain intact. Talc is a cheap filler in powders and mattifying lotions, and triclosan is a cheap antibacterial agent. Mineral oil adds viscosity so that the cream glides luxuriously on your skin. Many synthetic aromatic agents—sometimes as much as 200 of them in a single product—add beautiful fresh herbal or floral scents to otherwise blunt compositions.

When you choose between an unscented white fluid with uneven texture or a lavish iridescent crème that smells of violets and roses, what would you buy?

No matter what's the price, if you really care about your health, avoid carcinogenic ingredients in your skincare. The Body Shop and Urban Decay, for instance, are reformulating their product lines, taking out of their products chemicals linked to birth defects, and giving consumers safer choices. However, many companies continue using toxic ingredients in products bearing $100 and up price tags. Cynically, these products would be selling under a pink ribbon logo promoting breast cancer research. "They fight cancer by selling products that promote cancer," dryly noted Mylene, a sales associate behind a glittery cosmetic counter in Toronto.

Sad but true: many popular skincare products contain ingredients that pose certain harm to your health. This harm can vary from allergic reaction and minor rush to asthma, blindness and cancer. While it's almost impossible to eradicate all the chemical dangers from our lifestyle please use these potentially dangerous skincare products with great caution, and only for a limited time. We recommend that you never use skincare products with potentially carcinogenic ingredients when you are pregnant to minimize the risk for your unborn baby.

The best solution would be using products with unsafe ingredients for a strictly limited time, when you treat your acne, and then switching to natural organic skincare which is generally safer. Some plant ingredients and essential oils may also cause allergies, but frankly speaking, most people would rather choose allergies than cancer.

In the next chapters you will find a complete list of skincare recommendations designed for every acne-prone skin type. We will never recommend skincare products that contain carcinogenic ingredients. Each product we mention has been scrupulously checked for ingredients using safety data from reliable resources. You can find the complete list of such resources in the Appendix B.

To help you limit exposure to harmful chemicals in your skincare we will always recommend you a homemade natural solution that may not smell as good or packaged as nicely as commercial product, but homemade simple skincare will almost never increase your risk of having cancer or other serious disease.

From now on stop treating your skin as something separate from your liver, lungs or stomach. Skin is your largest body organ, and it's simply unwise to refer to it as to some kind clothes, something that you can only make look sexy and pretty, tan, smooth and shimmery. Skin is your vital organ that is tightly connected to the rest of your bodily systems, and unless you understand and accept it, you will never get rid of blemishes or skin irritations.

WHY ORGANIC?

The best way to avoid harmful or acne-triggering ingredients is to shop for organic skincare products. The best moderately priced brands to choose from are Avalon Organics, Kiss My Face, Weleda, and Jason Organics. More expensive options include brands such as Primavera, Lavera, Dr. Hauschka, Apivita (available in the UK and Europe) and Jurlique.

With so many "natural" products on the market, when even organic skincare manufacturers shyly label their products as "78% organic" stuffing them with parabens and triethanolamine, how can you possibly tell the real thing?

Some beauty manufacturers insist that there's no such thing as 100 per cent natural ingredient. Even when they distill essential oil or prepare beeswax people have to use chemically-enhanced machinery and unnatural tools made of plastic and metal, they say. For instance, cocoamide DEA is "derived from coconut oil." It comes from a perfectly natural source, so what's inorganic about it? Truth is, the manufacturing process of cocoamide DEA, just like many ingredients with DEA, TEA, MEA in their names, requires the use of carcinogenic synthetic chemical triethanolamine (TEA), monoethanolamine (MEA) or diethanolamine (DEA). So even if something comes from a natural source it doesn't mean it's organic and generally good for you. Just because vodka is made of wheat we don't consider it an organic remedy!

In the same time, chemical industry defines "organic" as any compound containing carbon. This makes methylparaben perfectly organic, as it was derived from crude oil, which is formed by leaves and animals rotting over millions years.

This is why cosmetic industry has developed the following definition of organic: this is a substance made of plant or animal which is grown, cultivated, and processed without the use of synthetic chemicals such as insecticides, herbicides, and fumigants. According to National Organics Standards Board, organic agriculture is an ecological production management system that promotes and enhances biodiversity, biological cycles and soil biological activity. Certified organic products are evaluated by third parties and comply with strict international standards which cover all aspects of the processing, from seed, harvesting, storage through the packaging of the product. Organic practices, however, cannot guarantee that products are completely free of residues, but organic methods help greatly minimize pollution from air, soil and water.

Advocates of synthetic high-end skincare often say that something natural doesn't mean it's safe and to prove this point remind you of some strong-smelling undiluted essential oils and irritating botanical extract such as peppermint or grapefruit. In fact, not a single organic skincare product we have purchased or tested for the inclusion in this book (and our team of organic beauty junkies tried nearly 500 of them!) caused any irritation that failed to disappear overnight. Organic beauty makers should make more concentrated lotions and potions—but this is just my humble opinion.

The bottom line is: anything you apply to your skin should be safe enough to eat. Whenever you put something on your skin, think: would I eat this? The reality is that anything you apply to your skin ends up inside your body just as if you had ingested it.

HOW TO BUY SKINCARE PRODUCTS

Fighting acne can cost you thousands of dollars, and for many of us, finding the right product we have to pass through certain period of trial and error. Every year hundreds of products claim to be the newest, the best and most effective treatments for acne. Acne sufferers constantly look for the magic lotion or potion that would turn their skin from bumpy to clear overnight and give us that flawless look we see on covers and pages of glossy magazines.

And since the cosmetics manufacturers are not likely to start cleaning up their acts anytime soon, your best bet to protect your health is to seek out pure and safe skin care products.

When choosing skincare products to take care of your acne-prone skin, you should always look at the product box or bottle. According to the new Canadian legislation, product labels must list all the ingredients regardless of their quantity. Often cosmetic manufacturers will separately list the concentration of the active ingredient, such as "2% lactic acid" and other helpful ingredients for your acne skin condition. If you are savvy enough, you would easily spot ingredients you should keep away from, as they may irritate your skin or worsen your acne by increasing oiliness. A good clean skincare product will be **free from petrochemicals, sulfates, synthetic fragrance additives, PEGs, propylene glycol, triethanolamine, diethanolamine, and parabens.**

However, sometimes even if you stumble upon a relatively safe and properly formulated acne treatment product, there's always something that can go wrong, and the search continues. Still, there are certain ways to minimize the money and time waste.

Always request a sample. Of course, most pharmacies don't carry sample sizes of $10 cleansers. To avoid disappointment, check the ingredients for possible irritants such as lemon oil, orange oil, grapefruit oil, or menthol, as well as harmful chemicals listed above. If you consider buying a skincare item from a department store, don't be shy to request a sample. Many private pharmacies will decant a small amount of cleanser or moisturizer in a clear jar.

Always return a product that gives you irritation. This way, you will un-clutter your beauty routine as well as indicate the cosmetic company (in a very remote way) that there's something wrong with their product. If drugstore refuses to refund, ask for the address of a company's headquarters or a local rep and return the product with an explanation.

Accept a store exchange if refund isn't working or you don't want to bother with returns. Take an organic substitute of a bothersome product if the store has it in stock, or take any sensitive skin product that you can use to calm down the irritation.

Read unbiased reviews on skincare boards and forums such as MakeupAlley.com. In most cases, the product that caused 75% of reviewers to break out will break you out, too. Same refers to redness, stinging or flakiness.

Read the label carefully. Watch out for commonly used skin irritating ingredients that do little to treat your acne yet can break havoc on your skin. You can find a list of harmful ingredients in alphabetical order in the appendix of this book. Print it and carry with you when you go shopping. You may also use the handy Shopping List feature at ewg.org—simply enter the features you expect from the product.

Opt for natural preservatives in your skincare. There are many gentle preservatives used in organic skincare products that prolong shelve life but do not disrupt your health: grapefruit seed extract, potassium sorbate, sorbic acid, tocopherol (vitamin E), retinyl (vitamin A) and ascorbic acid (vitamin C).

The best way to shop for skincare products is to become ingredient-wise. You have to stop being afraid of fine print and learn to read product labels to determine good and bad product ingredients, so that you can select skincare products that are most beneficial for you.

Here's how you can read through the fine print with ease. First pay attention which ingredient is listed fist. Good cleansers and toners start with water and glycerine in the beginning of the list, toners may begin with alcohol right in the first line. The general rule of thumb is: the higher amount of an ingredient the product contains, the higher position of it would be in the ingredients list.

For example, a bad toner would list a propylene glycol second in the list of ingredients; bad moisturizer will list mineral oil or petrolatum as its second ingredient, right after water. Such moisturizer will contain *a lot* of pore-clogging petrolatum and therefore will not be suitable for acne sufferers. However, a moisturizer that lists mineral oil somewhere in the middle of the fine print would less likely to cause breakouts but nevertheless is less suitable for oily skin than a moisturizer with no mineral oil at all such as a lotion based on light safflower or olive oil.

When you learn the trick of scanning the ingredients list for toxic chemicals and ingredients that can aggravate your acne, you will never purchase just because it looks pretty or elegant, thus falling prey of tricky advertisers and marketers. Once you've learned to read the ingredients label and identify marketing scams, you would be able to avoid wasting money and take a perfectly good care of your acne-prone skin.

START CLEANING UP YOUR ACT

We are careful about the water we drink, we choose organic and locally grown foods, but in fact the amount of chemicals we swallow with our food is very small compared to the amount of toxins we absorb through our skin.

Skincare formulated for problem skin is probably the most powerful ally in your battle against pimples. Cleansing gels dissolve grime and oil plugs in pores, astringent toners deliver acne medications right to the pore, and moisturizers help protect and heal. Unfortunately, many of these products are formulated with foaming agents linked to allergies, antibacterials potentially causing cancer, and preservatives ending up in breast tumors. In best case scenario, these ingredients will cause you allergies or new acne outbreaks. In worst case scenario, they will accumulate in your body triggering serious disorders.

Before we discuss skin care products that are most helpful for your acne condition and your skin type, let's take a look at products that we already own. This is the perfect time for you to edit your beauty routine and re-evaluate your beauty habits. Read the labels. Spot unwanted chemicals. Check the ingredients list and get rid of everything that contains one or more toxic ingredients that are listed in the previous chapters.

Many find that European cosmetics don't list as many toxic ingredients on their labels compared to similar products made in North America. This is because European standards are very strict, and many ingredients such as benzoyl peroxide are banned in European cosmetics. Even though many European skincare products are chemically-based, they are less dangerous to health. For example, a classic beauty product, Nivea Crème (made in Germany) doesn't contain parabens, triethanolamine or propylene glycol. And even though Nivea Crème contains mineral oil, this cream makes much safer choice for the protection of dry skin, especially in winter. My neighbor, 85-year old German lady, claims she has never used another cream in her life, and her skin is taut as an apple. Even least expensive European shampoos and conditioners, such as Fructis Garnier, will never contain DEA. They are not 100% organic, but still it's safer choice.

You don't have to throw out everything right away. Got a brand-new problem skin mask for $50 that lists triethanolamine on its label? Give it to your less picky friend or swap it online at one of beauty product swapping websites. Still can't part with that caviar-based moisturizer that is overloaded with parabens? Use it up as quickly as possible and replace with a lotion that is non-toxic.

Some "holy grail" beauty products are almost impossible to let go of. You may still keep a miracle hair balm if it does wonders to your hair and doesn't cause back or neck acne. However, we strongly suggest that you double-check all questionable products that sit on your skin for a long period of time, such as toners, moisturizers, and serums. Use them up quickly and replace with non-toxic versions.

Don't like the selection of cleansers and toners in health food stores? You can always find elegant organic formulations such as Dr. Hauschka, adored by Madonna and Jennifer Aniston, both famous for their glowing complexions, or Jurlique, also a favourite of many celebrities over 40. Other high-end organic brands include Lavera, Primavera, and Juice Beauty. There are also semi-natural skincare lines, such as Caudalie, REN Skincare, Weleda and L'Occitane that do not use parabens or chemical phenoxyethanol but do list a few safe chemicals on their labels. Most of these brands are available at Sephora stores or online. In the appendix C I list these brands along with places where you can buy them.

Another excellent source of new organic skincare lines is eBay where many spas have online stores. If you are open for things new and exotic, you can find amazing natural and mineral-based skincare from Iceland, Hungary and Israel, as well as herbs and clays for your homemade cosmetic creations. Always check the ingredients list or request one from the seller before buying anything.

If you don't have access or a budget to splash on Jurlique which has magic potions as pricey as La Mer or La Prairie I recommend trying simple affordable of homemade organic recipes suited for every skin type.

Keep in mind that when you switch to all-natural skincare your skin may start misbehaving. This is because many natural beauty products contain multitasking essential oils that work as spot treatments, anti-aging agents, and preservatives. Unless you become extremely allergic to one particular ingredient, so that you cough, sneeze and wipe tears, don't quit. In a couple of days your skin will adjust itself.

After revising your beauty stash, let's take a peek in your shower cabin. Most shampoos and conditioners, from less expensive Dove and Suave to salon brands such as Matrix and Sebastian contain petroleum-based ingredients, sodium lauryl sulphate, diethanolamine (DEA) or triethanolamine (TEA), as well as parabens. Unless you can't live without a particular conditioner, replace them all with organic versions or at least shampoos made in Europe such as Fructis by Laboratories Garnier. Dr. Hauschka, Prairie Naturals, Giovanni Organics and John Masters Organic make excellent hair care products, while Jason Organics makes sumptuous shower gels *sans* sodium lauryl sulphate.

Now that we are done with the bathroom, let's take a look at your makeup bag. By all means consider switching to mineral foundation, be it a compact or a powder. With a good quality mineral foundation (think Bare Escentuals) you get a decent buildable cover, an acne treatment, and a dependable SPF 15 that will be water-resistant, too. Later in the book we will share some professional tips on how to make mineral makeup work for you. Think about replacing your lipgloss or lipstick with a more pure version by Burt's Bees or Ecco Bella. An average woman eats half a pound of lip gloss per year, and you definitely don't need all those parabens and silicones in your stomach.

We don't expect that you will ditch all of your beloved, time-tested and quite pricey beauty treasures all at once. If your heart bleeds, put them all in one drawer and try switching to clean natural skincare for just one month. Give it a try. After one month, if you still feel like it, you can always go back to your chemical skincare. But something tells me that you won't.

HOW TO CHECK FOR INGREDIENT SAFETY

If you stumble across a perfectly natural lotion or a cream that makes perfect sense when it comes to treating acne, for example, based on olive and tea tree oils, some organic alcohol and astringent witch hazel, you may still find a couple of chemical ingredients which names you cannot pronounce. Sometimes these ingredients are safe to apply on skin, but sometimes it's worth checking twice, especially if your skin is sensitive or you are pregnant.

The complete up-to-date list of harmful toxic and potentially carcinogenic skincare ingredients based on Material Safety Data Sheet, FDA and Environmental Work Group reports can be found in Appendix A at the end of the book. Not many dermatologists and skincare retailers would agree with this list. Many would discourage you from, let's say, avoiding products with triethanolamine because they either are not aware of its danger or they have read ten-year-old report of FDA which states this product is safe **if not used in high concentration**. However, there's no evidence so far this product is safe when used in small doses over decades. This is why we encourage you not to take risks when it comes to your own health.

For each skin type and dilemma we will offer a few reliable skincare products commonly available in drugstores, department stores or online, at every price range, so you can follow our recommendations easily. We also suggest lifestyle, nutritional, and supplemental changes you need to make to take better care of your troubled skin. Your Skin Type chapter will also help you to pick products and procedures that are best suited for your particular skin condition.

With the detailed information about your acne-prone skin needs explained in future chapters, you can take control of your acne while staying on a budget. By following these tips and using your common sense, you will never end up buying products that go directly to trash or medicine cabinet, a "museum of ointments," as Jerry Seinfeld once said.

DAILY ACNE SKIN CARE ROUTINE

As you have learned in previous chapters, acne is caused by sebum and dead cells clumping together and sticking to the follicle walls as well as by the irritating effects of bacteria growing in the pore. We will try to reverse the acne formation process and stop the acne before it actually appears on the skin surface. The following skincare methods will also help your skin heal itself in its natural pace.

1. First, we will deep cleanse our skin to eliminate dirt and remove makeup;

2. Once a day, we will do a targeted skin treatment to eliminate skin cell buildup, soothe the irritated inflamed skin, or diminish scarring;

3. We will apply treatment toner on thoroughly cleansed skin to destroy the excess of acne bacteria;

4. We will apply a suitable moisturizer or a sunblock to help your skin heal faster;

In the next few chapters, we will explain how to take care of your skin in the right way and how to prepare and apply simple homemade solutions that have already made wonders to acne sufferers who have read the digital edition of "Clear Skin Guidebook." Later, we will talk about specific skin conditions and offer detailed step-by-step skincare guides for every skin type, such as young acne-prone skin, dark skin, mature skin and more.

How to Cleanse

Good acne skin care starts with the right cleanser. Some cleansers would simply rid the skin of accumulated sebum and remove makeup and daily dirt, whereas others will even our skin tone by exfoliating dead upper layers of the skin using tiny particles or alpha- and beta-hydroxy acids. For some people, acne starts improving once they master the art of the right cleanse. Surprisingly, it's very simple.

Here are essential technique for getting a really deep facial cleanse:

1. **Pick the right product.** There are many great cleansers available, from traditional foaming gels suitable for younger skin types, to cleansing milks and waters that do not later but work wonders for sensitive and mature skin types. There are newer types of cleansers such as self-foaming cloths and pillows that are both convenient and very effective. But, if your skin is dry and you suffer from acne, then keep away from cleansing creams that do not require rinsing, as they will block pores and increase the oiliness of infected area. **Remember**: you should avoid abrasive scrubs with scrubbing particles if you have acne flare-ups! Pimples should not be scrubbed as those tiny particles will break the protective cell layer and increase the inflammation. Exfoliating cleansers are useful when you fight brown spots left after acne blemishes have healed up.

2. **Use your fingers.** You should use only their fingertips for washing. Do not use any kind of sponge, Buf-Puf, or washcloths on the skin infected with acne for the same reason why you shouldn't use scrubs. Rinse your face with warm water and then pat dry. All this hardly takes a minute but makes a lot of a difference to your skin.

3. **Cleanse twice a day.** No matter if you have active acne flare-ups or you are working to prevent them, make a habit to wash your face once in morning and once in the evening. Wash or at least wipe your face after any vigorous activity which makes you perspire, like exercise.

4. **Morning cleanse should be gentle.** Work the cleanser of your choice in circular motions starting with your forehead and moving down to your cheeks and nose. Work the nose area well. Don't forget about your chin, throat and the jaw line area, especially under your ears. If you are using a medicated cleanser, for example, with salicylic or glycolic acid, leave it on for only a few minutes before rinsing.

5. **Double-cleanse in the evening.** In general, evening cleanse is more important than washing your face in the morning (which doesn't mean you can skip the morning wash!) Make it a new habit to double-cleanse in the evening. The first cleanse will rid of the surface dirt—airborne

particles, dust, makeup, sebum, residue from moisturizers and sun-blocks. The second wash, with cleanser containing clay, alpha- or beta-hydroxy acids will deeply cleanse your pores and deliver the acne zapper of your choice deep down where it's needed.

6. **Timing is everything.** Work your cleanser in circular motion for not less than one minute for regular morning cleanser and for one minute each step for a double cleanse in the evening.

7. **Rinse twice.** Rinse your cleanser thoroughly with lukewarm tap water and finish with a cool rinse, with tap, filtered or better yet, mineral water with essential magnesium such as Volvic, Vichy or Evian. Make sure to remove all of your cleanser: any soapy residue may clog your pores, cause blackheads, or further irritate already inflamed spots.

8. **Pat dry.** Gently pat your face with facial towel. Don't use your regular bath towel. Don't rub, either—this may cause unnecessary pressure and increase irritation. Be as gentle as possible.

Most people with acne think that frequent and vigorous cleansing with abrasive or antibacterial washes will reduce oiliness and help pimples heal faster. However, no scientific evidence proves that the lack of washing is associated with acne or that frequent washing improves acne. Instead, brisk cleansing and scrubbing can worsen the inflammation in acne breakouts, and antibacterial agents such as triclosan and chlorhexidine do not affect P. acnes. All they do is irritate your skin.

DO YOU NEED A TONER?

Initially toners were designed to remove the residue left on the skin surface after cleansing and deliver hydrating or soothing ingredients that remain on the skin surface. Since many people with dry or sensitive skin prefer using creamy cleansers that infuse skin with moisture, they don't need hydrating toners. On the contrary, people with acne-prone skin tend to rub their skin with irritating alcohol-based toner that contains "refreshing" peppermint and "pore shrinking" salicylic acid. All they achieve is additional irritation that only makes acne worse.

If you wash your face right and splash it with mineral water afterwards, you don't need anything else to remove the cleanser residue. There would be none left. What we do need is something healing and anti-inflammatory for our acne breakouts or something whitening and mildly exfoliating for post-acne marks.

There are few great toners that both soothe and heal, and we are going to prescribe them for each specific skin type. However, most sophisticated toners—I prefer calling them facial sprays or mists—are quite expensive and not always available, especially if you don't have Sephora nearby or your current budget doesn't allow splashing on precious organic finds at SaffronRouge.com. Here are some great recipes that work perfectly well on most acne-prone skin types. And they won't cost a fortune, too.

Homemade Skin Toner Recipes

Honey Tea Tree Oil Toner—All Skin Types

This toner works great to help heal existing blemishes and prevent new ones from erupting. Tea tree oil is the essential oil steam distilled from the Australian plant *Melaleuca Alternifolia*. Tea tree oil contains Terpinen-4-ol which is responsible for most of the scientifically proven antimicrobial activity of this essential oil. One of the most effective natural antibacterial treatments, tea tree oil is a natural antiseptic, which has been used for the last 70 years to treat skin infections, cold and flu, oral thrush, cold sores, gum infections, mosquito bites, herpes, sunburn and even vaginal yeast infections.

To prepare the toner we will need a 0.5 l bottle of Evian, Volvic, Avene or Vichy mineral water, some chamomile tea, organic honey, and vitamin C powder as a preservative and antioxidant.

1.   Drink half the bottle of water to make room for the rest of ingredients.

2.   Steep 3 packets of chamomile tea in a cup for 30 minutes. Pour the tea into the mineral water.

3.   Add five drops of tea tree oil, 1 tsp honey and a little bit of vitamin C powder as a preservative. Shake well until everything dissolves.

4.   Store the toner in a fridge, as you don't add alcohol or chemical preservatives.

5.   Use this toner in two weeks and prepare a new one.

If you are intimidated by the scent of tea tree oil, try Niaouli essential oil which is made of a similar plant, *Melaleuca Viridiflor*, which grows in Madagascar. Niaouli essential oil has same antibacterial acne-fighting properties, but smells less harsh and aroma is sweeter. You can use it in the toner just like the regular tea tree oil.

Rose, Witch Hazel and Vinegar Toner—Mature Skin

This toner is excellent if you are trying to get rid of post-acne spots. Rose helps soothe and heal the skin, while apple cider vinegar works as a gentle acidic peel dissolving and wiping away dead skin cells. Green tea is a known antioxidant that also helps prevent blemishes from reoccurring. To make the toner even more soothing and moisturizing you may add some chamomile in the mix.

To prepare the toner we will need a 0.5 l bottle of Evian, Volvic, Avene or Vichy mineral water, 3 packets of green tea, rose water or rose essential oil, and apple cider vinegar.

1. Drink half the bottle of water to make room for the rest of ingredients.

2. Steep 3 packets of green tea in a cup for 30 minutes. Pour the tea into the mineral water.

3. Add 3 drops of rose essential oil and 2 tsp apple cider vinegar. If you are using rose water, skip essential oil and add 3 tbsp of rose water in the mix.

4. Store the toner in a fridge—this way, you will always have a refreshing splash of deliciously scented herbal goodness!

5. Use this toner in two weeks and prepare a new one.

Apple Cider and Aspirin Toner—All Skin Types

Apple cider vinegar is helpful with it comes to lightening acne scars. To prepare an Apple Cider and Aspirin toner, dilute vinegar in the following proportion: eight parts water to one part vinegar.

1. Drink half the bottle of water to make room for the rest of ingredients.

2. Add apple cider vinegar to the top

3. Crush 5-7 aspirin tablets, add them to the toner and shake the bottle vigorously.

The potent combination of alpha-hydroxy and salicylic acids will make wonders to your skin—and this way you are not adding any chemicals or fillers. If you like the way it works, you can experiment with the concentration of apple cider vinegar in your toner. Some people swear by applying vinegar directly on skin, but this might be harsh for more delicate skin types. You can apply this toner directly to your skin with a cotton ball. Don't spray it in your face because it may irritate your eyes.

Aloe Vera, Lavender and Vitamin C Facial Mist—All Skin Types (Except Pregnant)

This facial spray feels great in the summer. You may spray it directly onto skin because it doesn't contain essential oils, vinegar or alcohol.

To prepare the toner we will need mineral water as above, 1 oz pure aloe vera juice (available in health food stores), lavender water or lavender essential oil, and vitamin C powder, also available in health food stores or pharmacies. We will also need a clean spray bottle.

1. Half-fill spray bottle with mineral water.

2. Add aloe juice and vitamin C powder. Shake well to mix.

3. Add 2 drops of lavender essential oil or 3 tbsp lavender water. Mix well.

You can store the toner in a fridge although it's not necessary unless you want to have a cooling spray handy. You may also decant the toner in a smaller spray bottle and carry it in your purse or gym bag for a quick refresher. Use this toner in two weeks and prepare a new one.

MOISTURIZERS

Many people with acne-prone skin types stay away from moisturizers. This is not the way to go: combination and even oily skin can lack moisture despite the oily shine on the surface. Besides, all skin types can benefit from soothing and nourishing botanicals, vitamins and minerals that many moisturizing lotions are packed with.

The key is to choose the right texture for your skin type. In general, oily skin can tolerate gels and gel-creams better. Combination skin benefits from lotions, and dry acne-prone skin can get all the help it needs from lightweight serums applied at night and in the morning under a sunblock. When the skin is very dry, products that come in creams or ointments are more appropriate. Sensitive skin types can well tolerate lightweight non-comedogenic evening primrose, rose and chamomile oils, applied under a sunblock or alone at night.

What to Expect from a Moisturizer

Perhaps the most important purpose of the moisturizer is to protect the skin from elements, such as UV rays, cold weather, and certain chemicals. When our skin becomes exposed to sun or harsh winds, sebum ingredients go out of balance, the skin becomes fragile, and outer skin cells are shed more rapidly. When skin balance is damaged, fragile inner layers of skin are exposed to outside irritants, which results in increased sensitivity. Skin becomes frail and prone to irritation which eventually results in acne.

Despite the name, moisturizers don't truly hydrate. We already know that delicate lower layers of our skin are protected from the outside world by a thick layer of keratinized dead skin cells. These cells and a layer of sebum work as a pretty resilient barrier. This is why no matter how hard you try to moisturize, cells beneath the top layer of the epidermis won't absorb any moisture. No matter how thick a layer of "revitalizing" mask you apply, flat dead cells of the skin won't come back to life. This layer of dead skin cells is quite water-resistant, too, so it won't let any of the active substances of masks and creams penetrate deep enough to the dermis layer to make any difference.

If you read the fine print on a skin lotion leaflet, you will see that cosmetic companies are quite aware of this fact. For example, they list the specific features of a cream, and note that it "moisturizes" with an asterisk. Then, the smart manufacturer will add somewhere in a less noticeable place that the product moisturizes "only the top layer of epidermis". This means that the cream will hydrate only those dead skin cells.

Of course, you need to moisturize the top layer of the skin to make it more pliable and look more attractive. If the moisturizer contains antioxidants and SPF, it will also protect your skin from elements. But moisturizing itself doesn't ward off wrinkles or sun spots. You can truly hydrate your skin only from within, drinking plenty of water, eating right and ensuring that your skin care products are emollient, not sticky, so they lubricate the top layer of the skin, not clog the pores.

However, keeping outer skin layer soft and healthy is vitally important. Outer skin layer, or skin barrier, determines whether your skin is dry or oily, sensitive or resilient, will it retain moisture or become clogged.

The following ingredients have been proven to soothe the skin and reduce the inflammation:

- Aloe vera
- Alpha lipoic acid
- Arnica
- Basil
- Calendula
- Carrot extract
- Chamomile
- Coenzyme Q10
- Copper peptide
- Cucumber
- Evening primrose oil
- Geranium
- Ginger
- Grape seed extract
- Green tea
- Lutein
- Lycopene
- Oatmeal (colloidal)
- Pomegranate
- Rosemary
- Silymarin
- Zinc

It's best to look out for a moisturizer that contains at least three of the above ingredients. In the next chapters we will suggest appropriate moisturizers, serums and masks for each problem skin type.

Why You Need Sun Protection

Sunscreen is a must if you have acne-prone skin. No matter if you spend your days lounging by the pool or working nine-to-five in an office, you have to wear a sunblock with at least sun protection factor (SPF) of 15—especially in the summer.

People who suffer from acne often shun sunblock for two reasons. First, there's a myth that sun helps "dry out" acne blemishes. Second, active ingredients in sunblocks are known to block pores and provoke blemishes, especially if your skin is already oily.

Nevertheless, sunblock have to become an essential part of your beauty routine. There's a plenty of scientific research proving that exposure to sun rays lowers the immunity in the skin making it more susceptible to infections and inflammation. Besides, when you expose your red swollen blemishes to sun they will leave dark brown spots behind. This happens because the skin in the inflamed spot produces melanin (pigment-producing) cells in bigger quantities, and when you expose inflamed unprotected skin to the sun, they produce more pigment, and the spot becomes darker with time. We all know that post-acne marks that are hard to get rid of. This is why prevention is your best tactic.

Many people with acne don't like sunscreen saying they are oily and increase breakouts or cause allergies. While some people can be allergic to chemical active ingredients in sunscreen, such as benzophenone, sometimes it's a vehicle that carries these ingredients that causes a problem. Try lightweight oil-free lotions or sprays with micronized zinc oxide if you have oily sensitive screen.

If you don't like layering products—and we don't blame you—choose only one multitasking product with an SPF 15. Pick a moisturizer with built-in sunblock or wear a hydrating serum topped with a mineral foundation that usually provides SPF 15 and higher. Don't forget applying separate sunscreen to your neck and upper chest which tends to age as fast as the skin under eyes.

Sometimes you may feel that sunscreen runs into your eyes and stings. If this happens, stop using a sunscreen around eyes. Instead, cover the area with mineral foundation or concealer or find a sunscreen that is approved for use in sensitive eye area.

Some dermatologists today don't advise to shun the sun entirely. First of all, sun is mood-enhancing, and the absence of sunlight is often blamed for seasonal affective disorder, mild mood disorder that is borderline depression and which is triggered by the absence of sunlight in winter months. Ultraviolet light helps increase the production of endorphins—the hormones that make you feel good.

Secondly, sun rays help "manufacture" vitamin D in the body. This vitamin has been shown to help protect against many deadly forms of cancer.

Sunbathing does have its benefits—but not for all skin types. People with darker skin tones—from olive to brown—usually tan well and rarely experience sunburns. However, keep in mind that repeated sun exposure can cause natural buildup of melanin which contributes to hyper-pigmentation in forms of brown spots in place of old acne scars. However, pigmented cells are known to protect cellular DNA and keep it from mutating into cancerous cells. But women with fair skin especially those with naturally blonde and red hair, should avoid sun and especially sunburn at all costs.

Even though moderate sunbathing does have its benefits, excessive "baking" in the sun not only damages skin's own defenses, it also speeds up aging by depleting collagen and weakening the supportive structures in dermis. This is why it's important to wear sunscreen marked at least SPF 15 or when in a sunny climate, an SPF of 45 and more, choosing the sunscreen with texture that suits your skin type. We will suggest best sunscreens for each problem acne-prone skin type in next chapters.

SCRUBS AND MASKS

Exfoliating your skin is essential. Exfoliating with alpha-hydroxy acids (AHAs) or tiny particles removes top dead skin cell layer and debris, promoting cell turnover and preventing pores blockages with dead skin cells and beauty product leftovers. Regular exfoliation also helps fade skin discolorations such as post-acne marks, and with time it may even help smooth more visible acne scars.

If you are working to prevent acne, you should exfoliate every day. Ideally an exfoliation with AHAs or a scrub should be followed by a clay- or charcoal-based mask that will deep-cleanse pores which you have already opened with a scrub. Here are a few sumptuous techniques to enjoy a spa-grade exfoliation and deep-cleansing at home.

Homemade Scrubs and Peels

You can exfoliate your skin using scrubs or acid-based masks and peels. Scrubs offer physical exfoliation using tiny synthetic or natural particles, such as jojoba or polyethylene beads, crushed walnut or grape seed. Alpha- and beta-hydroxy acids exfoliate by dissolving the very top layer of dead skin cells using glycolic acid from sugar cane, lactic acid from sour milk, tartaric acid from grapes, malic acid from apples, piruvic acid form citrus fruits. Malic and tartaric acids are more commonly used in exfoliating body products as they are more potent.

If you have inflamed acne lesions on your face or body, you should never use abrasive scrubs, no matter how natural or gentle they feel. Grain and beads in the scrub will further damage the fragile skin in the area of inflammation, so the irritation gets worse and all your efforts to speed up the healing process will go down the drain along with the scrub. Instead, use gentle exfoliating lotions and masks based on fruit acids.

Scrubs are best to use when you have no inflamed lesions but lots of post-acne spots or blackheads. You may use a scrub as a part of your daily double-cleansing routine as a second step following makeup-removing first wash. You can also use abrasive scrubs in your weekly home spa regimen before applying nourishing, whitening or deep-cleansing mask.

Baking Soda and Honey Scrub—All Skin Types

Baking soda is a very cheap cooking ingredient that you most likely have in your kitchen drawer. Baking soda makes a great scrub. Its fine particles gently rub off the dead and damaged skin, and it gradually dissolves on your skin, so there's no risk of damaging the skin or over-scrubbing.

Honey is an ancient remedy for the treatment of infected wounds. Ancient Greek healer Dioscorides described honey as being "good for all rotten and hollow ulcers." In laboratory studies, honey has been shown to have an antimicrobial action against many bacteria and fungi. Honey has healing and antibacterial properties thanks to low levels of hydrogen peroxide which are not dangerous during pregnancy or if you have an increased sensitivity to this ingredient.

When used fresh and undiluted honey penetrates deep into pores healing the inflammation. Some honeys have an additional phytochemical antibacterial component. For instance, the strawberry-tree honey of Sardinia is valued for its therapeutic properties; in India lotus honey is said to be a panacea for eye diseases; honey from the Jirdin valley of Yemen is revered in Dubai for its therapeutic properties; and manuka honey has a long-standing reputation in New Zealand folklore for its antiseptic properties.

To make a gentle yet powerful scrub, you have to mix 2 tablespoonfuls of baking soda with equal amount of honey to form a paste. If the honey is too dense you can warm it a little and it will become more fluid allowing mixing more accurate. Keep this scrub in a fridge for one week.

If you find that baking soda particles are too harsh on your freshly healed acne "leftovers" you can use oatmeal and honey for a very delicate yet effective scrub. Mix three tablespoons of plain uncooked oatmeal with three tablespoons of honey. This recipe has longer shelf life.

You can alter the Honey Scrub recipe and mix honey with green clay to create an absorbing and healing mask. You can apply honey directly on the face for a quick soothing treatment. Experiment with different sorts of organic honey to find out which one you like most.

Homemade Masks for Acne

Lemon Egg White Mask

Lemon juice is an excellent bleaching agent for minor facial discolorations, and it works as effectively as hydroquinone to lighten minor skin discolorations such as brown post-acne marks.

Egg whites are rich in protein and they help to heal and rebuild your damaged skin. Egg whites can also help to absorb excess oil from your skin.

Crack an egg, removing the yolk so that just the egg whites are left in shell halves. Beat these egg whites, and apply them directly to your face. Cut a fresh lemon in half and squeeze the juice into a shallow bowl. Mix in the egg whites and whisk to form a dense paste. Store this mixture in a fridge for one week and discard the unused portion.

Egg Whites Clay Mask

This mask works as a temporary lift while deep cleansing and drawing out impurities from the skin. It is most suitable for combination/dry skin.

In a bowl, mix 2 tbsp white clay and 1 tbsp corn flour. Beat in one egg white. Add 1 drop chamomile oil. If the paste is too thick, dilute the mixture with freshly brewed chamomile tea. Mix well to dissolve the egg white completely and apply on clean dry face. Allow to dry and wash off with tepid water.

Oatmeal Onion Mask

Onion acts as an anti-inflammatory agent and inhibits the overproduction of collagen in acne scars, while oatmeal penetrates deeply in pores cleansing the excessive cell buildup and pore clogging.

To prepare the Oatmeal Onion Mask, cook ½ cup of plain unsweetened oatmeal. Set aside to chill. Peel one medium onion and finely shred it in food processor making a smooth puree. Add it to the cooked oatmeal while it is still warm.

If the mask is not thick enough, add some honey or green clay until the mask is thick enough to sit comfortably on your face. Store the mask in a fridge for one week.

You may prepare all the toners and masks during the weekend and store them in a fridge for one week. Next weekend discard the unused portions and prepare a fresh batch.

Banana Honey Face Pack

This is an excellent reviving mask for tired lackluster skin. The mask is extremely easy to prepare and costs pennies.

In a bowl, mash 1/2 banana, add 1 tablespoon honey and 2 tablespoons sour cream (whole milk or skim-milk). Blend thoroughly so there are no clumps. Apply to face and let set for about 10 minutes. Gently wash off with warm water.

Strawberry Sour Cream Face Pack

This is a traditional European recipe that works wonders to breath life in dull dry skin. Strawberries are rich in vitamin C and sour cream contains lactic acid and proteins which both help to whiten post-acne hyperpigmentation.

In a bowl, mash 5-6 ripe strawberries together with 2 tbsp sour cream or fat-free cream cheese. Blend thoroughly so there are no clumps. Apply to face and let set for about 10 minutes. Gently wash off with warm water.

Cucumber Aloe Whitening Mask

Puree 1/2 peeled, sliced cucumber in a blender or food processor. Add 2 tbsp pure aloe juice, 1 tbsp powdered milk and 1 tsp honey. If the mask is too runny, add some kaolin clay until the mask forms a comfortably thick paste. Apply to clean dry face and leave on for 15 minutes or until dry. Gently wash off with tepid water.

Ultimate Whitening Mask

In this mask, antibacterial properties of honey are boosted with antifungal properties of lemon. Both lemon and yoghurt work as excellent natural peels helping fade post-acne marks. Egg white adds proteins that help strengthen skin's own defenses. You can store this mask in a fridge and use daily or every other day for one week.

Blend 2 tsp honey with 4 tsp lemon juice (freshly squeezed or bottled). Add 3 tbsp plain yogurt (approximately ½ small carton). Beat in 1 egg white and blend until all ingredients are well mixed. If the mask is too runny, add ½ tbsp kaolin (white clay) until you reach smooth creamy texture. Apply to clean dry face and let set about 15 minutes. Gently wash off with warm water.

Oatmeal Apple Cider Mask

This easy-to-make and wonderfully inexpensive mask doubles as a quick scrub and a deep cleansing treatment. Apple cider vinegar, rich in tannins and fruit acids, helps fade post-acne brown spots and soothe active inflamed blemishes. Grind 2-3 teaspoons raw plain oats in coarse paste. Add 1 tbsp honey and 1/4 teaspoon of apple cider vinegar (preferably organic) and blend until smooth. Add 1 drop of tea tree oil and blend more.

You can scrub your face with this mask or apply on a clean face to dry. Avoid the eye area. Leave the mask on for about 15 minutes and wash off with lots of tepid water.

ACNE TREATMENTS

Acne Home Facials

Even after you establish a healthy routine of daily double-cleansing, toning, treating and blocking sun rays, your skin needs a regular dose of high performance special treatment. Just half-hour a week can mean a huge difference! Here's a weekly facial routine that you can enjoy on a Friday night or Saturday morning. You can also admit your skin to the following intensive care if a sudden pimple pops up before an important event.

Wash your face with your regular cleanser. Rinse thoroughly with lukewarm water and blot dry with a fresh towel. Apply a homemade or organic exfoliant of your choice: a fruit acid-based peeling lotion if you have inflamed blemishes or a scrub with mild particles if you want to get rid of post-acne brown spots. Massage the exfoliant in circular motions for two minutes. Rinse clean and pat your face dry.

Prepare an anti-inflammatory facial steam bath: boil some filtered or mineral water, pour it in a ceramic, glass or metal bowl (careful: the bowl may get hot!) and add one drop of each of the following essential oils: chamomile, eucalyptus, rosemary and tea tree oil. Skip rosemary and use lemon oil instead if you are pregnant.

Cover your head with clean cotton towel and bend over the bowl. Let the vapors envelope your skin. Close your eyes and breathe slowly. Added bonus: your sinus condition will heal faster, too. Continue steaming for five minutes. When your face is still wet, apply another portion of a scrub and massage gently for two minutes. Rinse and pat face dry.

Apply a thin layer of a clay-based homemade or charcoal mask. Leave on until dry. Rinse clean with cool mineral water and pat face dry.

Apply your regular medicated toner and follow with a moisturizer.

The second technique is based on a totally different approach. Treat your freshly erupted pimples to this intensive procedure before an important event. First of all, wash your face with your regular cleanser. Rinse thoroughly with lukewarm water and blot dry with a fresh towel. Crack or crush several ice cubes and wrap them in a clean gauze or washcloth. Apply ice to the bump. Hold it in place for as long as you can stand the cold but no longer than 10 minutes. Remove the ice and dot on an over-the-counter acne medication containing lavender or tea tree oil. Repeat every four hours or so until the blemish has diminished in size and is no longer red.

Another emergency spot treatment works especially well if you have a painful highly visible zit and only five minutes to improve the situation.

Boil a cup of mineral or filtered water. Add a teaspoon of sea salt and make sure it dissolves completely. Make sure the water will not burn you. Saturate a cotton ball or gauze square in the mixture, press out excess, and apply to pimple for a minute or so. Now saturate cotton ball or gauze in witch hazel or rubbing alcohol and apply to pimple with very gentle pressure for thirty seconds. Blot dry.

Repeat these steps several times depending on how much time you have or until redness or oozing have diminished. If the pimple's white cap is removed during the steam/soak process, do not attempt to press out the contents. Continue salt compresses until the pimple is dry.

Popping Zits

Many dermatologists do not agree on the practice of squeezing zits. They believe that squeezing causes more infections and increased tissue damage—which is right if you squeeze the freshly erupted zit. If you look at the blackhead, they say, you see a solid lump of grease and a pigmented black cap on top of it. By squeezing this lump out, you might be clearing the pore, but you also risk pushing this sebum lump deeper inside, causing more damage that result in more scarring.

I completely agree that squeezing zits is a risky business. However, I have seen thousands of times when an average blemish left untouched would elope into a horrible volcano zit, painful and full of pus, which heals for weeks and leaves a horrible dark spot behind. I have also experienced zits that could be safely popped and the area healed perfectly within a day or two.

The decision to extract the acne pimple on your own should be done with care and knowledge. Here are some ground rules:

Rule #1. Wait until the pimple is fully developed on the surface and the white center is nearly bursting on its own. If you are trying to extract the reddish bump which has no cap and which is painful, you risk damaging blood vehicles nearby but you won't do anything to clear the pore of the blockage. You may also extract a blackhead if it shows a visible black cap and the skin around the pore is not inflamed.

Rule #2. Wash your hands thoroughly, especially the fingertips and under the nails, to get rid of any bacteria that could contaminate the already infected pimple. You may want to consider using sterile gloves or a gauze square. "It's best to keep your bacteria-laden hands away from your skin," dermatologist Alanna F. Bree, M.D., says.

Rule #3. Use right tools. Metal blackhead and whitehead extractor is the great tool to get rid of "ripe" acne and noticeable blackheads. This metal spoon is double-sided, with two metal loops on each side. The flatter loop is great to squeeze out whiteheads, the rounder smaller loops "forks" out blackheads and black stuffed pores around the face. The great thing about the loop is that is causes pressure right at the location of an acne spot, minimally damaging the nearby skin surface (unlike fingernails do.) Make sure to dab the spoon in alcohol before and after use.

Rule #4. Be cautious but be firm. Take a sterile, finely tipped needle and lance the center of the lesion. Next, gently squeeze the zit taking extra tissue from around the zit. Give equal amounts of pressure on every side. Continue until a clear liquid comes out. Use a clean, napkin, toilet tissue or gauze to dab away the liquid. Be careful not to spread it beyond the open zit.

Alternatively, you can use a medicine dropper. Position it so that the center of the pimple is at the hole in the dropper and the glass supplies pressure on all sides. Press gently until the pus is released.

Rule #5. Do not squeeze until you see the blood coming out of the zit! There's a sad myth that you should see the blood when you squeeze the acne: it means, some people think, that you reached the end of the pore and that the blood has washed away all the germs. This is a harmful deception! If you do see blood that means that you damaged the blood vessel beneath the hair root and this could potentially result in more inflammation and scarring. The pus that you are trying to squeeze has no live bacterium or any germs in it, everything live has been eliminated by your body's protectors, the white blood cells (macrophages). Hence, you are removing only dead matter, and there's no need to put that debris in your own bloodstream.

Rule #6. Allow some time to heal. If you were clean and gentle, pimple shaft should heal in a day or two. Leave it to dry without bandaging or covering. If there is swelling, you may want to apply a cold cotton disk moistened with grain alcohol, salt or witch hazel solution and hold it against the open zit for a few minutes.

If you have a stubborn zit that you simply cannot leave alone there are a few steps you can take to rush along its maturing process. First of all, prepare a mixture of 1/4 tsp. salt in about 1/2 cup of hot water. Then dip a gauze pad into the hot water and place the soaked cloth on your pimple or blackhead. Hold it there for several minutes. The heat should soften the blemish and draw the liquids to the surface. You may need to do it more than once. It is best not to squeeze until the white center is visible and appears to be ripe.

Pore strips can be effective in getting rid of some shallow pore clogging, but they are unable to clear away blackheads and ripe pimples. When we attach a pore strip on our nose and then tear away the dried strip, we all notice the dark globs of some pore substance. This is a sebum from the pore, not the blackhead. When we rip off the sebum off the pore, it is coming back—because that's just the way pores work.

MAKEUP AND ACNE

It's nearly impossible to avoid wearing foundation when you have an unsightly constellation of pimples, and I am not going to insist on you ditching makeup totally. Instead, I am going to share some makeup tricks that I learned working at fashion shows where models sometimes show up with full-blown zits resulting from hectic schedule, backstage stress, questionable diets, frequent travel and overabundance of not-so-healthy makeup they wear on a daily basis.

Many women are afraid to wear makeup because they worry it will make their acne worse. And this is actually true since the wrong makeup can make acne worse. There are two things happening to makeup after it is applied on skin. The powder or a blush either migrates into pores or comes off with physical friction, for example, when we touch our face or when we dress. Comedogenic effect occurs when makeup travels into the pore, it blocks the pore and the blemish formation begins.

However, better foundations and concealers can actually help unplug pores and improve the look of acne. A foundation with such ingredients as zinc oxide or vitamin C can help clear up acne faster. It can also provide protection from the sun's harmful rays. Alcohol, allantoin, kaolin, and titanium oxide help decrease the oiliness in the skin.

When you have acne, I suggest that you opt for a compact foundation such as MAC Studio Finish or mineral loose foundation such as Bare Escentuals' i.d. bare minerals but use it with your fingertips. This will allow you precise application and layering of the camouflaging product right where you need it. Choose products that have ten or fewer ingredients. If you prefer the look and feel of a traditional liquid foundation, look for ones that are based with silicones or nylons since this ingredient sits very smoothly on the skin and doesn't clog pores. Water-based foundations are made up largely of water with only a small amount of added oil which also decreases chances of new breakouts. Pore Minimizer Makeup by Clinique is an excellent example—it separates in the bottle and you need to shake it before applying, and it contains acne-fighting ingredients. Other decent foundations to try are The Supernatural Airbrushed Canvas Powder Foundation by Philosophy, Studio Fix by MAC, Infallible Makeup by L'Oreal (nylon-based) and Acne Results Foundation by Dermablend.

Makeup brush is a great tool, but not during the acne outbreak. First, even the softest Kabuki brush by Bare Escentuals applies an unnecessary pressure and scrubbing action on your healing flare-ups. Second, both natural and nylon bristles accumulate oil and bacteria, which can also be harmful. Same applies to sponges—stay away from those when you have acne.

Contrary to the popular belief, fingertips do not add oiliness to your skin—fingertips do not have oil glands! And if you carefully wash your hands prior to makeup application, you will get yourself the cleanest and most precise tool you could ever dream of. The next level of cleanliness and preciseness would be an airbrush machine, which allows an immaculate makeup application, but it can cost up to $400, not including special products.

Loose powder is another great way to mask skin blemishes and discolorations. It absorbs skin oil better than pressed powder which is great for oily-skinned users. Loose powder, mineral or not, is most effective if it is buffed into the foundation rather than patted.

It can be difficult to find the right blush without D&C red dyes which are highly comedogenic. Many women who wear wrong blushes on a daily basis have tell-tale arrays of acne pimples on their cheeks and cheekbones. If you absolutely need a blush, consider using a mineral blush or a lightly-hued blush applied very sparingly on top of the foundation.

Lipsticks, mascara and eye shadow are unlikely to cause or promote acne, although some lip glosses may clog pores around the lip line due to the presence of pore-clogging synthetic waxes or mineral oil. If you noticed that your lip area started looking bumpy with blackheads forming, toss the questionable lip gloss immediately. Blackheads around lips can be very painful but they heal fast.

Pimple Cover Up

Now is the trickiest part: covering the blemishes. The most potent concealers are made by MAC, Laura Mercier and Revlon in its Colorstay range. If you are slowly becoming an organic makeup junkie, do not fret: you are using only a tiny amount of a concealer, and whichever potentially toxic ingredients it contains, you are going to shield your skin with mineral foundation first anyway.

Before getting hooked on mineral makeup I enjoyed the flawless finish they provided, but while MAC and Laura Mercier have the most comprehensive color range, I found that staying power of Revlon Colorstay wand concealer allows me to perform the following trick.

Prep your skin with mineral foundation. Depending on a product of your choice, dispense a small amount of the foundation into the cap or in your hand and swirl the soft domed brush so that it absorbs enough powder. Shake the brush gently to get rid of excess. Less is more when it comes to mineral foundation, and you can always add another layer if you feel you need more coverage. Apply with round or criss-cross motion to cover the skin completely.

Never apply the camouflaging makeup with your fingers. Instead, use a thin synthetic brush. If you are using a cake or stick concealer, apply it with a clean eyeliner brush—make sure to wash it thoroughly before use or designate a special brush for concealing. Smallest artist's brushes work just as fine and they are less pricey.

Saturate the very tip of the brush with a concealer. Start applying concealer in circular motion starting at the center of the pimple, and work your way millimeter by millimeter. As you proceed, the quantity of the concealer on your brush diminishes, and you will blend the concealer easily. If you are using a wand concealer, don't apply it with the wand provided. You will contaminate the concealer and the brush with acne bacteria. Use the clean brush to grab the concealer from the wand.

Once you covered the zit with the concealer, dab some translucent powder or mineral foundation on top. Dust the spot with loose mineral powder or mineral foundation applied with clean eye shadow brush. Carefully blend the concealer if it's still visible with the surrounding skin tone. Voila! The concealer stays put all day long. You can use this technique with any decent concealer, and this way you can cover post-acne marks, too.

Don't tap your finger over the freshly applied concealer: you will never make large molecules of color to penetrate the skin, this is nonsense, but you will ruin your application for sure.

If you still feel you need more coverage, add a dot of a concealer on top of the foundation—and this time, don't blend. Remember that the dot should be covering only the spot and not the surrounding skin area.

Camouflage works best on skin that is in good condition. Before applying a concealer of your choice, cleanse and tone your face, but skip the moisturizer in the area of the pimple. Instead, treat the pimple with topical treatment such as tea tree oil or dot a tiny bit of milk of magnesia. This will help reduce redness and swelling and speed up the healing. If you wear foundation all over, apply it sparingly before concealing your blemish.

All-day maintenance of your camouflage is important. Don't pick, touch, or rub the blemish. Not only will this remove the careful work you've done, it can also promote the inflammation and may even cause oozing and swelling. If your face starts to shine, blot the skin with special oil-absorbent tissues or with a plain paper tissue.

Mineral Makeup How-To

Mineral make-up was developed about 30 years ago, but only recently won beauty world by storm. Many celebrities are already hooked: Courtney Cox insists that her makeup artists only use mineral foundation while prepping her for the movie filming, while Kathy Griffin and Daryl Hannah swear by Jane Iredale's anti-aging mineral makeup. So many brands have created their mineral foundations, seems like the traditional bottles will soon become obsolete. Just in the last few months Urban Decay packed sheer mineral powder foundation in their trademark purple jars (Surreal Skin Mineral Makeup), Laura Mercier is now offering Mineral Eye Powder eye shadows, and Cover FX created an eggshell-inspired futuristic bubble with mineral foundation and handy sponge.

Even though mineral foundation contains no oils or any organic additions whatsoever, some brands can't part with preservatives: philosophy stepped up with The Supernatural 4 in 1 Mineral Makeup SPF 15 (good) but packed the jar with parabens and phenoxyethanol (bad). Skin mineral makeup by New York makeup artist Alison Raffaele is very appealing when it comes to shades and packaging, but ingredients also include parabens.

No Sephora nearby? No worries! Drugstore brands are exploring mineral makeup, too, with Physician's Formula, L'Oreal, and Neutrogena now offering moderately-priced mineral makeup sets.

Mineral make-up usually comes in form of loose powder that can be used on face and eyes. Many makeup brands make multi-tasking mineral face colors that can be mixed together or added to clear lip glosses and even mascara for subtle color effects. Mineral makeup doesn't contain fragrance (other than delicate rose oil attar in Miessence line). Mineral makeup is also free of talc, alcohol, synthetic dyes, mineral oil or preservatives. This makes mineral makeup a perfect choice for women with acne, allergies, and rosacea. Mineral makeup can be used safely after microdermabrasions, lasers and chemical peels.

Another great thing about mineral makeup is that its fine texture allows for seamless blending into skin. No matter how many colors you layer, make-up is going to feel light and natural. By adding mica in the mix, mineral makeup gives the skin a dewy translucent radiance.

Mineral foundations and blushes usually contain ingredients that are very nourishing and healing for skin. While Bare Escentuals keeps their formulas pure and simple, using triple-milled minerals like titanium, zinc and mica, Jane Iredale adds pine bark and pomegranate extracts and even 24K gold for extra age-battling benefits. The newest and very promising direction in mineral cosmetics is mineral skincare pioneered by Bare Escentuals that offer night skin treatment in powder form.

Last but not least, mineral makeup multi-tasks working as a sunblock, acne spot treatment and color. Most mineral foundations contain natural UVA-UVB blocking agents such as titanium oxide and zinc oxide. Even if the product is not labeled with SPF 15 and up, rest assured it offers you a decent degree of sun protection. Among the best products in the range are Amazing Base Loose Minerals SPF 20 by Jane Iredale and i.d. Minerals by Bare Escentuals, Bare Naturale Mineral Makeup SPF 19 by L'Oreal and 4-in-1 Pressed Mineral Makeup Foundation by PUR Minerals.

Here are some basic tips on applying different kinds of mineral makeup:

Foundation: shake some mineral powder in your palm or a lid of a sifter jar and swirl the brush until all powder particles are tucked into the bristles. Then tap away excess: it's better to add more product later than apply a visible goop of a powder. Buff the powder foundation onto skin in circular motion staring on the outside of your face. Cover the cheek area and then work on your nose, forehead and chin. Add more powder until you are satisfied with the coverage.

Concealer: dry mineral concealers are more pigmented that foundations and can easily cover blemishes, broken capillaries, post-acne spots and even moles. Concealers can be applied directly on the skin or mixed into a thick paste with water or mineral makeup fluid such as D2O Hydration Spray by Jane Iredale.

Eye shadow: use your powder foundation as a base shadow and apply the color of your choice as a wash. You can add more details or intensity if you mix the eye shadow with water or mineral makeup fluid.

Blush: if there's one mineral product you want to try, this should be a mineral blush. Free from potentially toxic synthetic pigments and talc, blush can be used traditionally on cheeks or added to your lip gloss or lipstick for a perfectly coordinated look. To apply a mineral blush you would need a round soft brush with natural bristles or an artist's brush for pastels.

Lipstick: I have yet to find a perfectly mineral lip product without preservatives. However, there are some great natural lip balms but their color palette is still quite limited. Mineral colors help solve the problem. You can add mineral bronzer to your lip balm for a natural looking lip tint or brush a radiant mineral highlighter directly on your lips on top of a lip balm for a sparkly and very staying color.

ACNE SCARRING

To most people who suffer from acne, scars are even worse to deal with than pimples and cysts they originated from. Severe acne can lead to scarring in some patients, although not everyone tends to worry too much about them. Men are less concerned about acne scarring, which is sometimes considered a sign of masculinity. There are several Hollywood stars that made acne scars their trademark, for instance, Tommy Lee Jones or Brad Pitt. Many actresses, for example, Angelina Jolie, Jessica Simpson and Cameron Diaz, also bear post-acne marks, but carefully hide them under makeup.

Many people never get papules, pustules, nodules, or cysts because their follicle walls are strong and the pore is always forced open, creating a blackhead, before the wall can give way. Other people almost never get blackheads but have a lot of inflamed acne blemishes. This is because their follicle walls are not as strong. Unfortunately, there isn't much you can do to improve the condition of your follicle walls. You can't strengthen them up with special exercises or skincare products or vitamins. However, you can diminish the inflammation before it reaches the critical point damaging the pore and surrounding skin.

Why Do We Get Acne Scars

Post-acne marks and spots are an unfortunate byproduct of the immune system's successful battle against acne. Since an infected pore doesn't have room for all the white blood cells required to neutralize an infection, the surrounding area swells, stretching and tearing soft epidermal tissue to make room. Once the site of an infection has been cleared of infection, dead cells stockpile damaging the pore and surrounding skin structure. This results in a thickened layer of skin over the infection site (kelloid).

The most common type of acne scar is called "ice picks". These scars formed in place of cystic acne that affected deeper skin layers. If the dimpling of the epidermis tissue is slight, it will soon even out. If the scarring is deeper, you may need to consider some grade of skin resurfacing, either mechanical or chemical.

The second type of acne scars is called "craters" which form when a section of epidermis is trapped beneath scar tissue causing deeper pit. These pits can be wider, up to quarter-inch in diameter. These scars form when the acne is not severe and heals faster, so that body has no time to produce enough granulation tissue to fill in the wound.

In some people with thicker or darker skin, kelloid scars can form in the place of acne blemishes. These scars can be tender and even itchy; they are raised above the skin surface. Kelloid scars may grow in time if you add some weight, and they tan faster turning dark brown. Kelloid scars usually require treatment.

The most common approach to treating noticeable acne scars is to resurface the skin by such techniques as laser ablation, chemical peels, or dermabrasions. But most acne scars penetrate far below the level where skin can safely be removed. Only the most minor, superficial scars can actually be expunged. Most can only be reduced in size and depth. For optimum results depressed acne scars generally require both resurfacing and implanting cosmetic filler material such as collagen beneath the depression to raise it up.

You must remember that acne scar elimination is a lengthy process, and not all the scars can vanish completely. Even if you decide to try some radical measures, such as microdermabrasions, dermabrasions or chemical peels, it requires several sessions until you really see an improvement in your skin texture and tone.

Dealing with Post-Acne Marks

Most of the acne lesions that people call scars are in fact post-acne hyperpigmentation left after acne heals. The cells that make pigment, melanocytes, are located at the bottom of the epidermis. During the course of acne, melanin cells are passed onto other cells of the epidermis and make their way up to the top layer of skin forming the dark spot. Usually this happens when the blemish was forced to "pop" or when the area was burned with potent alcohol- or salicylic-acid based topical treatments leaving it open to sun rays and elements.

In any case, it's important to remember that these marks are not scars and require no treatment. Most of these marks can be covered by makeup, and will eventually fade, most often in three-four months. This process can be accelerated with various procedures. Among more natural solutions are home peels with glycolic acid, a powerful sugarcane derivative which exfoliates the outer layer of the skin, diminishes the darkness and stimulates collagen production. To soothe the skin, you can use reparative and calming masks and moisturizing lotions.

Before we deal with post-acne hyperpigmentation, or brown marks, make sure that your acne is completely gone. Most treatments for scarring will perform some degree of "damage" to skin, even though only the thinnest top layer of skin will be removed or bleached. You surely don't need this kind of irritation while acne bacteria still lurks in your skin.

To prevent acne marks and scars from happening never pick on your acne blemishes and never try to squeeze the pimple if it's not ready. Once an acne lesion is traumatized, it will take longer to heal and will be more likely to leave behind a mark. This is especially true if you have acne in the older age. A lesion that can heal in days in a teenager can take weeks or months to resolve in a woman over 40 and can still leave red or brown marks.

Sometimes your skin may be more genetically prone to forming post-acne dark marks. Usually, people with dark hair, fair skin, and an excess of birthmarks and moles are more prone to suffering from dark spots after acne is healed. People with fair skin and blonde or red hair often note that their post-acne marks remain red for a long time before they either clear up directly or finally turn brown, while people with olive or darker skin tones and dark hair note that they only get some pigmentation which fades away within weeks.

Most often, post-acne dark spots are treated with lightening creams—many of which contain extremely toxic substances.

Mercury salts were once a mainstay of skin bleaching, but they are almost obsolete today due to the high toxicity of mercury. Medical reports describe patients with high levels of mercury poisoning among patients in Mexico, Saudi Arabia, and Senegal, as well as Bosnian and Albanian refugees in Germany. Most of the patients with clinical evidence of mercury poisoning were women. In every case, doctors found that the women had used mercury-based skin-whitening creams for long time.

Another dangerous bleaching agent, hydroquinone, kills off the pigment-producing cells of the skin. However, this ingredient has been found to be extremely toxic and even carcinogenic[51]. The European Union banned hydroquinone from cosmetics in 2001, but it shows up in nameless bleaching creams in the developing world. Hydroquinone is still sold in the United States and Canada as an over-the-counter drug. Perhaps the reason why hydroquinone is so popular is that this chemical is extremely cheap. In Thailand hydroquinone sells for about $20 per kilogram (2.2 pounds), compared with natural (and much safer) licorice extract, which sells for about $20,000 per kilogram.

There are many natural ingredients that help lighten the skin without risk of cancer or other adverse side effects. Mulberry extract, abovementioned licorice extract, yeast ferment, rosmarinic acid, glucosamine, vitamin C, and chamomile extract are known for their whitening and melanin-inhibiting properties. Kojic and azelaic acid are well-studied and effective natural whitening agents favored by many dermatologists.

Whitening Treatments to Fade Acne Marks

Whitening ingredients work in two ways to prevent and diminish post-acne dark spots as well as other discolorations of your skin. When applied on top of the acne blemish they absorb the UV rays preventing the darkening the inflamed area. They also reduce the production of melanin, the skin pigment found in your skin which is responsible for skin darkening.

Here are some of the ingredients you may find in your skin whitening products:

Kojic acid used to lighten the skin in Japan. Kojic acid is a by-product in the fermentation process of malting rice for use in the manufacturing of sake, the

Japanese rice wine. Kojic acid works by inhibiting the activity of tyrosinase, which is the essential enzyme in the biosynthesis of the skin pigment melanin. Kojic acid is used in concentrations ranging from 1-4%. Although effective as a skin-lightening gel, it has been reported to have high sensitizing potential and may cause irritant contact dermatitis. In a study comparing kojic acid with hydroquinone, no difference in efficacy was reported, however, the kojic acid preparation was reported to be more irritating and less toxic than hydroquinone. Kojic acid contains in many commercially available skin-whitening treatments, including Pigment of Your Imagination SPF by philosophy, Lancome Skincare by Lancome Blanc Expert XWII Extra Whitening Spot Corrector, and Potent Botanical Skin Brightening Gel Complex by Peter Thomas Roth (unfortunately, all these products also contain triethanolamine, parabens, and other chemical toxicants).

Licorice extract has been used in Europe since prehistoric times, starting with the ancient Greeks. Licorice (*Glycyrrihiza glabra*) contains glycyrrhetinic acid, a powerful depigmenting agent that inhibits the production of melanin. One research shows that licorice extract slows down cancerous tumor growth and could prove useful in protecting some forms of human cancer. Licorice extract is used in Precision Performance Anti-Taches Roll-On treatment by Chanel and natural Antioxidant Recovery Treatment C by Boscia.

Alpha hydroxy acids are known for their ability to lighten skin discolorations by dissolving the very top layer of skin. Alpha hydroxy acid products will not inhibit melanin production by themselves, but when combined with licorice extract or kojic acid they help these ingredients penetrate the skin better and increase their effectiveness. Alpha hydroxy acid peels, done at home or in dermatologist's office, also show great results.

Chinese herbs, especially water extract of Galla Chinensis and ethanol extract of Radix Clematidis, may decrease pigmentation by causing lower tyrosinase activity in skin. Chinese scientists obtained potential skin whitening agents from 90 traditional Chinese herbs[52]. Nine herb extracts were proved to have depigmentation activity similar to or better than that of arbutin and low toxicity. However, studies have been carried out only in lab, and not on humans.

Salicylic acid peel is a particularly effective treatment for both acne and post-inflammatory hyperpigmentation that are common in patients with darker skin tones. During a well-documented study in South Korea, patients had undergone full-face peels with 30% salicylic acid in absolute ethanol bi-weekly for 3 months. No other topical or oral treatment for acne was used during the study. As a result of two-week treatment, 88% of the patients noted moderate to significant improvement, while only 16% experienced minimal to mild side effects[53]. Doctors say that salicylic acid peels may be especially effective in whitening post-acne marks in Asian and Hispanic patients with acne.

Glycolic peels have also proven themselves as a great option for darker skin that bears post-acne marks. There are many glycolic peel home kits available, such as Neostrata Skin Rejuvenation System, Neutrogena Advanced Solutions Facial Peel, or DDF 7 Day Radiance Peel Kit. Glycolic acid peels are also effective for melasma and fine facial wrinkling. Please note that during the course of peels you will have to use a sunblock with minimum SPF 15%.

Topical **vitamin C** (ascorbic acid) is one of the most readily available topical skin whitening treatments. Vitamin C has been proven to normalize dark melanin cells, reduce inflammation that leads to dark post-acne marks, and encourage collagen production. To effectively lighten skin tone, vitamin C must be in high concentration and freeze-dried. Vitamin C needs to be protected from elements and bacteria to preserve its potency. That's why only few products that pack vitamin C in mono-doses or in ready-to-mix fresh skin treatments truly deliver results. A randomized, double-blind, vehicle-controlled Canadian study involving women aged 36 to 72 who used topical ascorbic acid in Cellex-C high-potency serum made by Cellex-C International shows impressive 84% improvement in skin tone and elasticity after 3 months of treatment. The great thing about vitamin C is its safety and preciseness: you can apply it topically and intensively on your post-acne marks or you can treat the whole face with vitamin C serums. There are many quite effective formulations with vitamin C available on the market, and we will recommend appropriate treatments for each skin type in further chapters.

Vitamin B3 (niacinamide) is another vitamin that has been proven to lighten the skin color when topically applied. It also improves the tone and elasticity of aging skin. During a well-documented study women aged 50 and up were using 5% niacinamide (vitamin 3) serums for one month. All of them reported the decrease of hyperpigmented spots and overall skin sallowness. Among the most effective treatments containing vitamin B3 on the market are Advanced Signs Treatment and LXP Activating Massage Fluid made by Japanese high-end skincare line SK-II.

Arbutin is a glycosylated hydroquinone found at high concentrations in certain plants. Like hydroquinone, arbutin has been shown to inhibit melanin synthesis but it does not hydrolyze to liberate hydroquinone. That's why arbutin has been shown to be less effective skin whitening agent—and less toxic one—than synthetic hydroquinone. However, it also has antibacterial properties and has been shown to calm down skin allergies. This ingredient is used in Arbutin White

Cream by DHC, Revital Whitening Lotion and Whitess Intensive Skin Brightener by Shiseido and in mineral concealer Enlighten Concealer by Jane Iredale.

Although an effective topical concentration for treating disorders of hyperpigmentation has not been formally evaluated and published, several manufacturers are marketing arbutin as a depigmenting agent. Several studies have shown that arbutin is less effective than kojic acid for the treatment of hyperpigmentation. Some manufacturers report arbutin as an effective whitening agent at a 1% concentration.

Azelaic acid is a naturally occurring saturated dicarboxylic acid distilled from plant *Pityrosporum ovale*. Azelaic acid has also shown to inhibit of tyrosinase and kill melanocytes to help whiten skin. Initially azelaic acid was prescribed for the treatment of acne, but it is also helpful with rosacea and post-acne hyperpigmentation. Azelaic acid is prescribed topically as a 20% cream and has been combined with glycolic acid (15% and 20%). This combination has been shown as effective as hydroquinone 4% cream, but azelaic acid may cause more irritation. On a positive side, it's less toxic than hydroquinone, and side effects are also scarce. Azelaic acid contains in Potent Skin Lightening Gel Complex by Peter Thomas Roth (which also lists hydroquinone as one of gel's ingredients) and Recovery Treatment Gel by Murad.

When you have active acne blemishes or trying to get rid of their unsightly residue, remember that staying out of the sun as much as possible is necessary to prevent hyperpigmentation and skin aging. In summer, use a good sunscreen and don't overindulge in sun bathing.

TAKING CARE OF ACNE-PRONE SKIN

To work on your acne problems you have to treat your skin with respect. This means you need to know when it needs more water and when it needs more oil, or just when it has to be left alone to let it recuperate and heal itself. The only way to do it is to know your skin type.

We are not going the traditional way and offer you skincare tips for oily, dry and combination skin. Skin types can change greatly with seasons, diet, age, or health conditions such as pregnancy or menopause. So we are going to offer you skin care suggestions for teenage acne-prone skin, for acne-prone skin in young women, for dark and Asian skin, men, pregnant women and newborns (yes, they get acne sometimes, too!) and for mature acne-prone skin type. So even if you know your skin type—say, combination/oily,—you can reassess it depending on the season or changes in your lifestyle.

For example, if you have taut oily skin in your 30s, feel free to browse "Acne in Teenagers" chapter for a quick fix. If you feel you need some nourishment, go ahead and check "Acne in Mature Skin" chapter. Treat your husband or a boyfriend with some pampering tricks from "Acne in Men" section, and suggest a tip or two to your coworker who is blessed with lovely ebony skin but often feels helpless battling pimples along her hairline.

Feel free to experiment and explore—and feel safe to do it, because we tested all of our recommendations on ourselves and our trustworthy clients and friends. Please note that all products mentioned in the next chapters do not contain or contain a very minimal amount of synthetic or potentially toxic ingredients.

ACNE IN TEENAGERS

For some reason acne shows its ugly face in our teenage years when we especially need to feel confident and look good. The very origin of the word "acne," or *acme,* in ancient Greece meant "point or peak" or puberty, which was then considered to be the peak of life. And today acne peaks in young women between the ages of 14 and 16, when their hormones kick in, and in boys between the ages of 12 and 17. Early teenage acne usually shows up as blackheads and whiteheads around the center of the face and on the forehead. Later in puberty, inflammatory lesions are common.

These are the most common qualities of teenage acne-prone skin:

- Your skin is taut and firm with healthy glow
- You don't have crows feet or sun damage
- Your skin never feels tight, even after a cleansing with foaming gel cleanser
- Your skin looks shiny, sometimes as fast as 20 minutes after you washed your face
- Your t-zone (nose, forehead and chin) always have visible blackheads
- You develop acne blemishes at any time of the month
- Your acne blemishes usually heal within a week

Many parents believe that teenage acne is simply an age-related rite of passage that does not need to be treated because their child will "outgrow" it sooner or later. However, acne can be a very serious condition that would make a deep impact. If left untreated, teenage acne can result in scarring, low self-esteem and emotional problems. Because teenagers are minors, parents also need to be educated and encouraged to take their teenager's acne very seriously.

Luckily, there are many easy, natural and not expensive ways to treat acne. In your teenage years, skin is very resilient, taut and oily, and your face may often look shiny. Skin's oiliness and active hormones can lead to acne which may leave post-acne hyperpigmentation and scars. Sometimes you may overindulge in mattifying moisturizers, stinging cleansers and strong alcohol- and acid-based toners. This eventually leads to increased sensitivity, new breakouts and faster skin aging due to moisture loss.

This is why you need a consistent and effective yet gentle skincare routine. If you act to prevent breakouts and establish your own skincare ritual, you'll find that you can successfully prevent many skin problems later, in your 30s and beyond.

General Guidelines for Teenage Acne-Prone Skin

- Wash your face with a non-foaming or light-foaming water-soluble cleanser that does not sting or leave skin feeling dry.

- Cleanse only twice a day. Frequent or vigorous cleansing will increase irritation and inflammation but will not promote healing of your acne blemishes.

- Choose a toner that contains witch hazel, tea tree oil, plant-derived alcohols and clay, either bentonite or kaolin.

- Begin using a night treatment for acne that promotes healing and calms down the irritation. Choose fluids and serums over oil-free moisturizers.

- Make sure you wear sunscreen, especially in the summer or when you have active breakouts. Mineral sunscreen is perfect for young acne-prone skin: you can wear it on top of your acne treatment of choice.

- Exfoliate daily, with alpha/beta hydroxy acid product if you have active acne breakouts and with scrubs if you have no blemishes but want to fade post-acne hyperpigmentation.

- Start wearing an eye cream or lotion rich in antioxidants, vitamins, and water-binding moisturizing agents. Choose products that are packaged in airtight pump containers to keep the ingredients stable.

- Devote at least half-hour every week to deep cleansing skin treatment and oil-absorbing mask. With homemade masks you don't have to spend a lot of money.

- Develop organic consumer habits by reading ingredient lists and avoiding potentially toxic chemicals that may affect your hormonal balance and result in more acne. If you eliminate hormone-disrupting chemicals early you may avoid many devastating health disorders, including polycystic ovarian syndrome, and you will have better chances for a healthy pregnancy later in life.

Top Five Things to Avoid

- Don't cleanse too often and don't over-scrub your face. Too much pressure may lead to more pimples as your skin gets irritated and inflamed with constant mechanical pressure.

- Avoid greasy, sugary foods, as well as carbonated drinks and too much caffeine. Treat yourself to some ice cream and candy only occasionally—as a reward for good skincare habits during the week!

- Don't try to dry out your blemishes with toothpaste or other drying solutions. Really dry top layers of skin can trap impurities and bacteria under skin making acne worse.

- Don't pile makeup on your acne blemishes. Wear a concealer where needed. Use oil-blotting papers to absorb the excess shine during the day.

- Don't pick at your face. Keep your hands off the pimple until it's ready to be extracted and never attempt to pop up a tender red blemish. If you have time, try one of the procedures described in the previous chapter, and apply a topical antibacterial product containing salicylic acid or tea tree oil.

Daily Skin Care Plan

Morning:

- Remove the night treatment and refresh the skin with lightly foaming cleanser.

- Refresh the skin with toners and astringents that contain natural acne healing substances.

- Apply a topical treatment on acne blemishes

- Don't forget about sun protection to prevent the formation of post-acne brown marks. Apply a mineral foundation or lightweight mineral sunscreen, especially in the summer.

Evening

- Double-cleanse to remove makeup, sunscreen, and daily grime.

- Soothe and heal acne blemishes with a magnesium mask. To quickly soothe inflamed acne lesions and prepare your skin for a healthy night sleep apply a milk of magnesia for a few minutes before going to sleep. Use unsweetened unscented Magnesium Hydroxide—the common laxative and upset stomach treatment—straight on the face, leave it to dry and wash off with tepid water.

- Instead of a moisturizer, supercharge your skin care ritual with intensive nighttime acne treatments.

- It's never early to prevent aging of delicate skin around eyes. Use lightweight eye cream to restore eye freshness at night. You can also use a good moisturizer without SPF around your eyes.

Recommended Cleansers

$ Aveeno Clear Complexion Foaming Cleanser
$ ZAPZYT Acne Wash with Soothing Aloe & Chamomile
$ Burt's Bees Orange Essence Facial Cleanser
$$ Origins Checks and Balance
$$ DHC Mild Cleansing Soap
$$ DHC Deep Cleansing Oil
$$$ Jurlique Tea Tree Foaming Facial Cleanser

Recommended Toners

$ Thayers Original Witch Hazel with Aloe Vera
$ Aubrey Organics Blue Green Algae Facial Toner
$$ Burt's Bees Garden Tomato Toner
$$ Biotherm Pure Bright Refreshing Clarifying Toner
$$$ Dr. Hauschka Skin Care Clarifying Toner

Recommended Topical Treatments

$ Miessence Organics Purifying Blemish Gel
$$ Benefit Boo Boo Zap!
$$ Aveda Outer Peace Acne Relief Lotion
$$ Philosophy On A Clear Day Blemish Serum
$$ Boscia Willow Bark Breakout Treatment

$$$ N.V. Perricone M.D. Pore Refining Concealer

Recommended Sunscreens

$ Aubrey Organics Blue Green Algae Moisturiser SPF15 (for oily skin)
$ Aubrey Organics Natural Sun SPF 20 Tinted Sunscreen (for combination skin)
$$ Dr. Hauschka Sunscreen Lotion SPF 15 (for normal/dry skin)
$$ Bare Escentuals i.d. bareMinerals Foundation SPF 15
$$$ Jane Iredale PurePressed Base SPF18

Recommended Night Treatments

$ Miessence Organics Purifying Blemish Gel
$$ Boscia Willow Bark Breakout Treatment
$$ Jurlique Rosemary-Sage AHC
$$ Jurlique Pine Needles AHC
$$ Suki Facial Moisture Serum with Blue Chamomile and Echinacea
$$$ Jurlique Herbal Recovery Mist

Recommended Eye Creams

$$ Living Nature Firming Eye Gel
$$ Bare Escentuals bareVitamins Eye Rev-er Upper
$$ Korres Natural Products Yellow Hibiscus Eye Serum
$$$ MD Skincare Continuous Eye Hydration

Recommended Masks

$ Aubrey Organics Blue Green Algae Soothing Mask
$$ Origins Clear Improvement
$$ Jurlique Moor Purifying Mask
$$$ Dr. Hauschka Facial Steam Bath followed by Cleansing Clay Mask

Lifestyle Suggestions

Taking care of your skin as early as possible doesn't end in your bathroom. Maintaining a proper diet, exercise routine and managing stress are all important elements in your acne skin care challenge. You should also avoid acne triggers, such as humidity and heat. In summer or when in hot climate make sure you drink a lot of water and have a refreshing facial mist to cool down your skin. Remember that sunburns, hot wax depilation, peels, and strong chemicals can irritate your skin and lead to acne. Close-shave razors increase the risk of developing ingrown hairs, which also can increase inflammation.

ACNE IN YOUNG WOMEN

Graduating from high school doesn't necessarily mean the end of acne drama. According to Johnson and Johnson research, 71% of women aged 25 to 49 years old say they have had acne in the last year. And even though acne doesn't cause the same psychological trauma to grown-up women as it did to them in teenage years, the mechanism of acne and its origins are technically the same. While most women manage to achieve clear, smooth skin by the age of 30, most of them suffer from deep-seated painful zits that appear approximately a week before the period. These zits are caused by premenstrual shifts in hormones which prompt sebaceous glands to excrete more oil. In some women, hormonal influences sometimes don't take effect until 20s or 30s and occasionally even later in life. Chronic stress doesn't help, either.

Acne that occurs in young women often shows up in different places than it does in teenagers. Adult acne tends to center more on the lower part of the face, around the chin, and along the jaw line. This is why adult acne can be more difficult to control because the skin in this area is more sensitive.

Now, as your skin evolves into a new stage, your main focus should be acne prevention, not just treatment. Most likely, you are suffering acne since your teenage years, and past outbreaks have left lots of post-acne brown spots and maybe even scars. To fade them and prevent new acne blemishes from happening, you should use a daily exfoliating product, either a moisturizer or a mask. Don't forget about a sun protection that would help prevent premature aging and post-acne hyperpigmentation. Prevent premature aging and inflammation by strengthening your skin's own defenses by enriching your daily skincare regimen with antioxidants, vitamins and anti-inflammatory substances.

General Guidelines for Adult Acne-Prone Skin

- Make sure you thoroughly remove makeup using double-cleanse technique and non-foaming cleansers with exfoliating particles if you have no inflamed lesions or non-cleansers with fruit enzymes, clay or AHA if you have active breakouts.

- Avoid drying acne medications that can dehydrate your skin and lead to premature aging.

- Choose a toner that does not contain alcohol but is packed with chamomile, aloe, cucumber, calendula and fruit acids to gently exfoliate the skin.

- Wear a daily moisturizer with anti-oxidants such as vitamin C, green tea, tocopherol, grape seed extract, gingko biloba, Echinacea, beta carotene, Avena Sativa (oat) and superoxide dismutase. All these ingredients will protect your skin from free radical scavengers.

- At night, use a serum or a lotion packed with botanical anti-inflammatories such chamomile, green tea, panthenol, provitamin B5, tocopherol (vitamin E), licorice, calendula, raspberry, rice, oats, seaweed (algae), evening primrose oil, arnica, and Echinacea.

- Regular exfoliation with botanical enzymes such as papain (papaya enzyme), bromelain (pineapple enzyme) and alpha- and beta-hydroxy acids will dissolve dead skin cells and help fade post-acne hyperpigmentation.

- Invest in a good eye cream that fights and prevents signs of aging as well as protects delicate eye area from the environment. Look for ingredients such as vitamin A, C, E, peptides, panthenol, vitamin K (for dark circles), and bioflavonoids. Choose products that are packaged in airtight pump containers to keep the ingredients stable.

- Take a daily dose of vitamins and antioxidants with additional alpha lipoic acid and omega 3 fatty acid supplements.

- Hone your organic consumer wisdom by reading ingredient lists and avoiding potentially toxic chemicals that may affect your hormonal balance and result in more acne. If you eliminate hormone-disrupting chemicals early you may avoid many devastating health disorders later in life and you will have better chances for a healthy pregnancy which you might already be planning.

Top Five Things to Avoid

- Don't skimp on water. Drink 7-8 glasses of mineral or filtered water a day. Don't replace water by carbonated sugary drinks and coffee. Remember your skin is the largest organ of your body and is the first to become dehydrated.

- Avoid or at least diminish iodides in your diet because they can aggravate your acne. Iodides occur in seafood, kelp products (seaweed), beef liver, soy sauce, MSG, turkey and asparagus.

- Don't overindulge in sunbathing. Aside from being the number one cause of skin cancer and pre-mature aging sun also increases your skin's oiliness resulting in more pimples.

- Never go to bed without removing your makeup!

- Don't use at-home microdermabrasion or peels more frequently than once a week. Too much scrubbing and peeling results in increased skin's sensitivity and acne.

Daily Skin Care Plan

Morning

- Remove the night treatment and refresh the skin with non-foaming cleanser with gentle scrubbing particles, fruit acids or enzymes.

- Gently exfoliate with a toner containing plant enzymes, alpha- or beta-hydroxy acids.

- Apply a topical treatment in a form of serum or light lotion.

- Apply a moisturizer that provides protection from sun and free radicals. Wear a mineral foundation or lightweight mineral sunscreen, especially in the summer.

Evening

- Double-cleanse to remove makeup, sunscreen, and daily grime.

- Finish the cleansing with a toner to remove the cleanser residue and calm down your skin.

- Soothe and heal acne blemishes with a magnesium mask. To quickly soothe inflamed lesions and prepare your skin for a healthy night sleep apply a milk of magnesia for a few minutes.

- Supercharge your skin care ritual with intensive serums. Apply a vitamin C powder directly on blemishes. To treat larger areas affected with acne mix with 1 scoop of philosophy Hope and a Prayer vitamin C with 2-3 drops of your favourite facial or body oil. Vitamin C will not dissolve completely. Please note: this concoction may sting.

- Delay and repair premature aging of eye area with intensive eye cream.
- Every other day: homemade scrub followed by a homemade mask to promote healing and fading of post-acne hyperpigmentation.
- Every week: a home microdermabrasion or a home peel.

Recommended Cleansers

$ Desert Essence Tea Tree Oil Facial Cleansing Pads
$ Earth Science Clarifying Facial Wash
$$ Origins Never A Dull Moment
$$ Dr. Hauschka Cleansing Cream
$$ Suki Lemongrass Cleanser
$$ Primavera Refining Exfoliating Cleanser
$$ LUSH Fresh Farmacy Skin Cleanser
$$ Jurlique Face Wash Cream
$$ DHC Mild Cleansing Soap
$$ DHC Deep Cleansing Oil (for double-cleansing)
$$$ Dermalogica Precleanse (for double-cleansing)

Recommended Toners

$ Aubrey Organics Natural AHA Fruit Acids with Apricot Toning Moisturizer
$ Aubrey Organics Green Tea and Gingko Facial Toner
$ Caudalie Grape Water
$$ Caudalie Beauty Elixir
$$ Dr. Haushka Clarifying Toner
$$ Origins Oil Refiner
$$ Pangea Italian Green Mandarin with Sweet Lime
$$$ Zirh Refresh

Recommended Moisturizers/Sun Protection

$ Aubrey Organics Green Tea and Ginkgo SPF 15 Moisturiser
$ Trevarno Organic SPF 15 Day Cream
$$ Bare Escentuals i.d. bareMinerals Foundation SPF 15
$$ Dr. Hauschka Sunscreen Lotion SPF 15 (for normal/dry skin)
$$ MD Formulations Total Protector 30
$$ Juice Beauty SPF 30 Tinted Moisturizer
$$$ Korres Watermelon Sunscreen Face Cream SPF 30
$$$ Jane Iredale PurePressed Base SPF18

Recommended Topical Treatments

$$ Origins Grin from Year to Year (spots)
$$ MD Formulations Vit A Plus Clearing Complex (acne, spots)
$$ philosophy Prayer in a Bottle (acne, spots)
$$$ Juice Beauty Antioxidant Serum (spots)

Recommended Night Treatments

$$ Aubrey Organics Sea Buckthorn with Ester-C Rejuvenating Antioxidant Serum
$$ Primavera Wild Rose Face Oil Capsules
$$ Jurlique Ultra Sens Night Treatment Gel
$$ Philosophy When Hope Is Not Enough
$$ Suki Facial Moisture Serum with Blue Chamomile and Echinacea
$$$ Dr. Hauschka Rhythmic Night Conditioner
$$$ Jurlique Herbal Recovery Gel

Recommended Eye Creams

$ Aubrey Organics Lumessence Rejuvenating Eye Crème
$ Weleda Wild Rose Intensive Eye Cream
$$ L'Occitane Olive Oil Express Eye Treatment
$$ Dr. Hauschka Daily Revitalizing Eye Cream
$$ Boscia Enlivening Amino-AG Eye Treatment
$$ Ecco Bella Eye Nutrients Cream
$$$ Emerita Fine Line Eye Serum, Multi-Peptide Complex
$$$ Jurlique Eye Gel

Recommended Peels

$ Neutrogena Advanced Solutions Facial Peel
$$ MD Formulations Alpha Beta Daily Face Peel
$$ Juice Beauty Green Apple Peel—Full Strength
$$$ Kinerase Instant Radiance Facial Peel
$$$ Fresh Appleseed Resurfacing Kit

Lifestyle Suggestions

Stocking proper skincare products is important for proper skincare, but developing good habits is even more vital. To avoid acne from reoccurring, eat the right foods and de-stress any way you can. Start practicing yoga and meditation if you haven't already. Cut down on caffeine and alcohol, drink lots of water, and stick to organic food whenever possible. If you have to buy non-organic fruits and vegetables, focus on avocado, bananas, broccoli, cauliflower, kiwis, pineapple, pineapple and watermelons, as these products contain least pesticides. Get a multivitamin loaded with antioxidants and take an additional supplement containing omega-3 fatty acids.

Visits to spa can be great for your skin but remember that hot wax depilation, peels, and strong chemicals can irritate your skin and lead to acne. Close-shave razors increase the risk of developing ingrown hairs, which also can increase inflammation. You should also avoid such acne triggers as humidity and heat. In summer or when in hot climate make sure you drink a lot of water and have a refreshing facial mist to cool down your skin. Avoid rigorous sunbathing and wear sunscreen to prevent the formation of dark spots. Whenever you notice a suspicious growing mole, immediately see a dermatologist.

As you continue managing pigmentation and overactive oil production, you may wish to explore stronger treatments, such as lasers and intense pulse light treatments. They can improve your skin condition greatly.

Coping with problem acne-prone skin requires some effort, but over time, you'll come to understand your skin's behavior. Oily/combination skin is a mixed blessing: it requires constant upkeep, but in future you have more chances to delay or even bypass costly anti-aging treatments.

ACNE IN MEN

For most men, skincare is similar to shoe shopping: they *honestly* don't get what's all the fuss. Contrary to popular belief, acne is just as common among men of all ages as among women. Young men are especially likely to suffer from acne for longer periods of time because high levels of testosterone stimulate the sebaceous glands to produce more oil than necessary and make acne worse. However, most men are not going to read this book—just like they would never spend much time and money buying cleansers, toners, and eye creams—which means that it's up to us, women, to share these bits of acne-fighting knowledge with men in our lives.

Luckily for them, most male acne sufferers have natural built-in mechanism that prevents them from getting severe acne and post-acne hyperpigmentation. Male skin is thicker, oilier and more resilient, and their acne tends to heal faster and flawlessly. In addition to that, the daily shaving routine acts like a thorough skin scrub followed by an antibacterial treatment with aftershave, which already contains acne-fighting ingredients. However, when acne is present, shaving is a real pain. Men rarely want to switch their tested-and-true shaving foams and aftershaves that often cause breakouts and razor burn. Shaving can also cause ingrown hair and skin irritations which aggravate the existing acne condition.

Below you will find some useful tips on how to shave safely while preventing acne. Battling acne doesn't have to involve many bottles and tubes, and you can always borrow a trick or two from the chapter on acne in young women.

Remember, acne is easier to prevent than to get rid off, and in case of acne in men, organized grooming with only few carefully selected products will help men take care of their skin more efficiently.

General Guidelines for Treating Acne-Prone Skin in Men

- Invest in a pre-shave skin cleanser that will prep the skin better than any irritating pre-shaving solution. The cleanser may be lightly foaming, scented or non-scented, gentle and water-soluble.

- Buy shaving products that are non-irritating and contain as less chemicals as possible. Traditional foaming shaving creams are known to cause less razor burn than shaving foams and gels.

- Not using the right blade can cause acne by constantly abrading the skin and causing micro-cuts that get infected. Buy your man a good-quality shaving blade as a gift or a reward for something special. Practice shows that men genuinely avoid buying skincare products until their shaving foam canister is empty, but they almost never resist a gift.

- Replace an aftershave with a toner—lots of cosmetic brands make toners that are fairly unisex and non-scented or naturally-scented.

- Most men use soap to cleanse their faces. If your man has fine and sensitive skin, think about replacing his soap (most likely, a plain soap bar) with a stylish chunk of Marseille olive soap that doesn't contain irritating and drying ingredients.

- Find a good moisturizer, preferably unscented, that your man would use with dignity. Avoid golden caps, floral scents, and frilly packaging design. Before buying a new skincare item, ask for a sample and give it to your guy to try.

- To help your man combat aging buy him a moisturizing lotion with alpha- or beta-hydroxy acids. This lotion should be used only in the areas that are not shaven daily—for example, on the forehead, nose and around eyes. Warn your man not to apply the lotion on freshly shaven skin.

- We still have to see a man that would allow us to slap a clay mask on his face. Still, men are becoming more open to using scrubs. Invest in a face polisher that contains natural jojoba beads or other plant-based scrubbing particles.

- Make sure your man takes his dose of antioxidants, vitamins and minerals specifically formulated for men with lutein, lycopen and alpha-lipoic acid.

- Practice stress relief together whenever possible. Day-to-day stress that occurs in the workplace and in your personal life is known to build up and affect your health including hormonal and immune systems. Stress also causes the body to produce an excess of hormones, which in result cause the man to break out. Massages, yoga for couples, exercise can work wonders in helping your man unwind.

Top Five Things to Avoid

- Avoid shaving products that form thick foam—they always contain sodium laurel sulphate and similar ingredients that can cause skin irritation which many men mistake for razor burn.

- Don't use aftershaves that burn, sting or make your skin red. Avoid ingredients that are known to irritate the skin. These ingredients include alcohol, menthol, peppermint, eucalyptus, lemon, lime, and camphor.

- Using old blade will not only burn, it will also spread bacteria infecting micro-cuts and nicks.

- Picking pimples has never made anyone look good. Men are more likely to attempt squeezing their zits until blood shows. Vigorous squeezing can cause post-acne hyperpigmentation (dark spot) that may stay tender really long partly because of daily shaving.

- Overindulging in drying acne medications can only worsen the situation. A topical treatment containing tea tree oil or salicylic acid applied directly on zits—and not all over the face—should be just enough.

Anti-Acne Shaving Technique

- Shaving starts the typical man's day. However, it's best to avoid shaving right after the awakening. It's best to shower first allowing the puffiness in your skin diminishing. This will help you shave more closely and safely.

- Before shaving, wash your face with a cleanser to open up the pores of the skin and prepare it for a close shave. Some men find that shaving in the shower makes their skin more hydrated and pliable.

- Wet the face with water as hot as you can tolerate before shaving. This swells the hair shaft allowing the blade to cut the hair, not your skin.

- Choose a thinner, lightly foaming shaving cream that helps the razor glide effortlessly over the skin. A plant-based shave cream, not foam, will provide a close soothing shave and help you avoid nicks and razor burn. Massage the cream thoroughly into your face working into a thick protective lather.

- Use a sharp blade. A blade is too dull if it drags or catches your skin along with the stubble. If you are prone to acne and ingrown hair, use a single-blade razor. Newest multiple-edged blades promote ingrown hair by lifting the stubble out of the follicle and cutting the hair below the epidermis. When the epidermis grows, it closes over the opening of the follicle, so the hair is trapped under skin's surface. However, if ingrowth continues, as it sometimes does in curly haired men, consider switching to an electric shaver.

- To prevent a buildup of shaved hairs from interfering with clean shaving, rinse the razor frequently as you work.

- Shaving with grain means shaving in the direction of how the hair grows on your face. Usually it means you should shave down. Shaving up, or against the grain, can cause redness, rashes, razor burn and ingrown hairs, which are all painful. However, men with dark hair and fair skin sometimes have to double-shave. In any case you must never shave over active inflammatory acne lesions. Don't shave over pustules.

- If you prefer using an after-shave, choose an alcohol-free toner to avoid dryness and stinging. Avoid any aftershave products that leave cooling sensation. This means they have irritating menthol, peppermint or eucalyptus among their ingredients. Pick a toner that contains aloe vera, witch hazel or tea tree oil instead.

- After shaving, apply an oil-free moisturizer with SPF to soothe and protect the face.

Recommended Shaving Creams

$ Aubrey Organics Men's Stock North Woods Shave Cream
$ Weleda Shaving Cream
$ Living Nature Soothing Shaving Cream
$$ Korres Natural Products Absinthe Brushless Shave Cream
$$ Anthony Logistics for Men Shave Cream
$$ Living Nature Gentle Shaving Cleansing Gel
$$ Zirh Shave Gel
$$$ Jurlique Men's Herbal Shaving Gel

Recommended Aftershaves/Toners

$ Avalon Organic Botanicals Hydrating Toner
$$ D'Arcy Original Drying Lotion
$$ Dr. Hauschka Clarifying Toner
$$ Aveda Outer Peace Acne Relief Lotion
$$ Weleda Shaving Lotion
$$ Weleda After Shave Balm
$$ Tend Skin
$$$ Zirh Refresh
$$$ Jurlique Men's Herbal After Shave

Recommended Moisturizers/Sun Protection

$ Aubrey Organics Green Tea and Ginkgo SPF 15 Moisturiser
$ Weleda Men's Facial Moisturizer
$$ MD Formulations Total Protector 30
$$$ Jurlique Men's Herbal Antioxidant Moisturizer

Lifestyle Suggestions

Make it a habit to use sunscreen marked at least SPF (sun protection factor) 15 daily, no matter if you plan to surf or spend your day in the office cubicle. UVA harmful rays go through windows in cars, buildings and airplanes. Choose sun protection based on titanium dioxide, it helps control oil.

In general, if you have acne, keep your skin care regimen simple and use carefully selected products to help control and prevent future breakouts. All the other aspects of healthy anti-acne lifestyle that we've discussed earlier in the book, from diet to stress relief and exercise, apply just as fine to men as to women.

ACNE IN SKIN OF COLOR

Taking care of acne-prone skin of color skin is very challenging. More pigmented skin complexions—those of South Asians, Native Australians, African-Americans, and Caribbeans—have an increased amount of melanin in the skin. Pigment cells are larger in people with darker skin, and they cover a greater proportion of the skin protecting it from sunlight and keeping people with darker skin looking younger than Caucasians. In fact, black people have a natural sun protection factor of 13, new study shows.

Unfortunately, large content of melanin also causes darker skin to be more prone to excessive and uneven pigmentation. As black people age, their skin often becomes irregularly pigmented. Irregular pigmentation caused by acne and sunburns shows up as dark patches on the skin. Black people almost always get a post-acne dark spot after the acne heals! This is why anyone with dark skin must stay away from all ingredients that cause inflammation and trigger acne. Common antioxidant vitamin C, anti-aging AHA and alpha lipoic acid, at-home peels and microdermabrasions can also spark an inflammation in darker skins. This means that many common acne treatments such as salicylic acid are also a major no-no, as well as common hair removers like Nair and hot wax depilatories.

If you have post-acne hyperpigmentation, microdermabrasion and topical bleaching may help fade excessive pigment more quickly. However, young black people who are being treated for acne usually have a reaction to the drying and peeling acne medications. The discoloration can last for years further promoted by lotions and creams that contain the drying ingredients. This is why you should avoid harsh scrubbing and abrasive treatments as they can cause inflammation in other areas while treating the darker spot. Never pick the pimple—picking and incorrect squeezing is a sure-fire way to post-acne scars and marks! Acne scars can be really devastating in darker skin. In case of severe acne darker skin is prone to forming kelloid scars which are extremely difficult to treat.

Another distinctive quality of black skin is the ashy tone that develops if the skin is lacking moisture and sheds dry skin cells too quickly. Darker skins need heavy oil-based nutritive creams that penetrate deep into the skin preventing it from looking dull and ashy. Besides, if not nourished properly, darker skin tends to loose elasticity very easily. However, we know that heavy creams and butters can clog pores and start the vicious acne cycle. In dark skin, acne may show up as many tiny bumps that don't look inflamed but in fact are typical acne with bacteria and sebum trapped beneath skin's surface.

So what's a girl to do if she has acne? Luckily, with a few carefully chosen products you can prevent and heal those nasty pimples that ruin your otherwise great—and ageless—complexion.

General Guidelines for Treating Acne-Prone Dark Skin

- Make sure you thoroughly remove makeup using double-cleanse technique and gentle non-foaming cleansers. Don't scrub or chemically peel your face if you have acne blemishes.

- Avoid using whitening agents all over your face. This can lead to uneven pigmentation and ashy, grayish complexion.

- Choose a toner that does not contain alcohol but is packed with chamomile, aloe, cucumber or calendula to gently exfoliate the skin. Avoid fruit and glycolic acids as they can promote inflammation.

- Wear a daily moisturizer with non-irritating anti-oxidants such as green tea, tocopherol, grape seed extract, gingko biloba, Echinacea, beta carotene, Avena Sativa (oat) and anti-inflammatory ingredients such as camphor, melissa, tea tree oil, panthenol, provitamin B5, tocopherol (vitamin E), and humectants such as Hyaluronic acid, honey, and sodium PCA.

- At night, use nourishing skin oil that will not clog pores. If your skin is dry, you can wear it under a day moisturizer, too.

- Remember to always wear your sunblock. Try to buy an elegant and appealing sun protection moisturizer that you would enjoy wearing. Most Black women don't realize is that regardless of the amount of pigment in your skin, long term exposure to ultraviolet rays means a higher risk for melanoma—much higher than in lighter Caucasian skin colors. Make sure to check your skin regularly for any unusual spots or moles.

- Regular exfoliation with gentle natural skin buffers—oatmeal, jojoba beads,—will eradicate dead skin cells without triggering inflammation.

- Invest in a good eye cream that fights and prevents signs of aging as well as protects delicate eye area from the environment. Look for ingredients such as peptides, panthenol, vitamin K (for dark circles), and bioflavonoids. Choose products that are packaged in airtight pump containers to keep the ingredients stable.

- Take a daily dose of vitamins and antioxidants with additional alpha lipoic acid and omega 3 fatty acid supplements to keep your skin glowing.

- Hone your organic consumer wisdom by reading ingredient lists and avoiding potentially toxic chemicals that may affect your hormonal balance and result in more acne. If you eliminate hormone-disrupting chemicals early you will avoid many devastating health disorders.

Top Five Things to Avoid

- Don't use heavy hair pomades or hair oils around your hairline. They will clog pores around your forehead and cause pimples. Too much hair pomade can aggravate seborrhea, an inflammatory, scaly, itchy skin problem.

- Don't use drying or peeling acne medication as they can cause uneven pigmentation that can last for years.

- Try not to scratch your skin if you have allergies. You may develop allergies to hair dyes; dyes in leather and nickel in earrings. Scratching can trigger acne reaction in skin.

- Don't mistake moles caused by seborrheic keratosis for acne. These moles are usually brown or black raised, dark spots that appear on the cheeks. These are not cancerous, but many women prefer to remove them.

- Don't use hair treatments for corn-rowing, hot combing, and hair-straightening chemicals close to hairline. These too can lead to skin irritation and acne.

Daily Skin Care Plan

Morning

- Remove the night treatment and refresh the skin with a non-foaming cleanser or natural olive oil soap.

- Gently refresh the skin and remove the cleanser residue with toner that doesn't contain alcohol, AHA or exfoliating enzymes.

- Apply a tea tree oil treatment on acne blemishes.

- Apply a moisturizer that provides protection from sun and free radicals. Wear a warm-toned mineral foundation or lightweight mineral sunscreen with a bit of golden shimmer, especially in the summer.

Evening

- Double-cleanse to remove makeup, sunscreen, and daily grime.

- Finish the cleansing with a toner to remove the cleanser residue and calm down your skin.

- Soothe and heal acne blemishes with a magnesium mask. To quickly soothe inflamed lesions and prepare your skin for a healthy night sleep apply a milk of magnesia for a few minutes.

- Replenish moisture in your skin with skin oils.

- Delay and repair premature aging of eye area with an intensive eye cream.

- Every other day: gentle homemade oatmeal scrub followed by a home-made mask to promote healing and reducing post-acne hyperpigmentation.

Recommended Cleansers

$ Kiss My Face Olive & Green Tea Bar Soap
$ Australian Organics Pure Plant Soap, Evening Primrose Oil
$$ philosophy on a clear day
$$ Jurlique Face Wash Cream
$$ DHC Mild Cleansing Soap
$$ DHC Deep Cleansing Oil
$$$ Dermalogica Precleanse

Recommended Toners

$ Kiss My Face Flower Essence Toner
$ Aubrey Organics Green Tea and Gingko Facial Toner
$ Caudalie Grape Water
$ The Body Shop Tea Tree Oil Toner
$$ Suki Concentrated Facial Toner with Shitake, Burdock and Olive Leaf
$$ Caudalie Beauty Elixir
$$ Dr. Hauschka Clarifying Toner

Recommended Moisturizers/Sun Protection

$ Aubrey Organics Green Tea and Ginkgo SPF 15 Moisturiser
$$ Bare Escentuals i.d. bareMinerals Foundation SPF 15
$$ Dr. Hauschka Sunscreen Lotion SPF 15 (for normal/dry skin)
$$ MD Formulations Total Protector 30
$$$ Korres Watermelon Sunscreen Face Cream SPF 30
$$$ Jane Iredale PurePressed Base SPF18

Recommended Face Oils

$ Kalaya Emu Oil
$ Weleda Almond Face Oil
$$ Eleusian Rosehip Regenerative Face Oil
$$ Primavera Evening Primrose Oil
$$ Dr. Hauschka Normalizing Day Oil
$$ Dr. Hauschka Translucent Bronze Concentrate
$$$ Jurlique Day Care Face Oil
$$$ Primavera Ultra-Rich Energizing Seed Oil Capsules

Recommended Eye Creams

$ Aubrey Organics Lumessence Rejuvenating Eye Crème
$ Weleda Wild Rose Intensive Eye Cream
$$ L'Occitane Olive Oil Express Eye Treatment
$$ Dr. Hauschka Daily Revitalizing Eye Cream
$$ La Fleur Organique Anti-Aging Eye Cream
$$ Suki Eye Repair

Lifestyle Suggestions

Reducing stress is extremely important, especially because dark skin is prone to specific stress-related skin condition called lichenification. It's harmless but unpleasant byproduct of nervous scratching. People who are under constant stress often develop itchy areas—back of neck, forearms, legs and ankles, and other areas—that they (naturally) scratch and rub. This condition leads to hyper-pigmentation which is very hard to get rid of. Practice anti-acne stress relieving procedures, exercise daily and eat balanced, preferably organic diet with little dairy to reduce your exposure to synthetic hormones. Get a multivitamin loaded with antioxidants and take an additional supplement containing omega-3 fatty acids.

You should also avoid such acne triggers as humidity and heat. In summer or when in hot climate make sure you drink a lot of water and have a refreshing facial mist to cool down your skin. At home, try to increase the relative humidity to at least 40 percent to prevent ashy skin complexion. At the same time, avoid sunbathing during midday and wear sunscreen to prevent the formation of hyper-pigmented spots. Whenever you notice a suspicious growing mole, immediately see a dermatologist.

Coping with dark acne-prone skin requires some effort, but over time, you'll come to understand your skin's nature. Please remember that many problems of dark skin are related to cosmetics and fashion trends that are more common among black men and women. Black skin is a mixed blessing: is can be very high-maintenance but it will reward you with glowing wrinkle-free complexions for many years to come.

ACNE DURING PREGNANCY

Pregnancy is the most exciting period in woman's life. The body undergoes so many changes, it's hard to imagine everything is going on by itself, without us even knowing it. And along with the excitement and anticipation there are also a few discomforts and ailments. Acne is one of them. It's not as distressing as nausea and constipation, but it may add up to mood swings, and when accompanied with widening waistline and heavy breasts, it can seriously undermine even the healthiest of self-esteems.

Acne usually shows up in the first trimester of the pregnancy, gets worse by week 16 and in most cases disappears by week 24. It can appear in women who has never had acne before. Sometimes women who were suffering from acne for years may find that their skin has wonderfully cleared up by itself. All skin changes during pregnancy are caused by major hormonal shifts. Higher levels of androgen hormones prompt the sebaceous glands in your skin to increase the production of sebum, which sooner or later leads to the inflammation and acne. Hormone fluctuations may also stimulate excessive pigmentation. If you have acne, the post-acne pigmentation may linger for longer time, and new moles and spots may also appear, especially if you have darker skin or very dark hair and fair skin.

Acne treatment is tricky during pregnancy because none of the traditional medications can be used. Both chemical acne treatments—such as salicylic acid—and natural remedies, including essential oils and fruit acids are not recommended during pregnancy.

General Guidelines for Acne-Prone Skin during Pregnancy

- Cleanse your skin with a pure olive oil soap or non-foaming natural-based cleanser. Avoid scrubbing your skin if you have an acne inflammation. After washing, pat your skin, not rub. Don't use washcloths or Buf Pufs.

- Choose a toner that does not contain alcohol but is packed with chamomile, aloe, cucumber, calendula to soothe and calm your skin.

- Wear a daily moisturizer with anti-oxidants such as vitamin C, green tea, tocopherol, grape seed extract, beta carotene, Avena Sativa (oat) and honey. All these ingredients will protect your skin and won't harm your baby.

- At night, use a serum or a lotion packed with botanical anti-inflammatory agents such chamomile, green tea, panthenol, provitamin B5, tocopherol (vitamin E), calendula, raspberry, rice, oats, seaweed (algae), and evening primrose oil.

- Regular exfoliation with homemade scrubs or face buffers with jojoba beads will dissolve dead skin cells and help fade post-acne hyperpigmentation.

- Fatigue and sleeping problems can make you look tired. A good eye cream will revive the eye area. Look for ingredients that either are natural or occur naturally in human skin such as vitamin C, E, evening primrose oil, panthenol, green tea, or elastin and peptides.

- Take a daily dose of prenatal vitamins. Ask your doctor if you should take an additional calcium supplement and fish oil (not fish liver oil!)

Top Ten Things to Avoid

- Avoid the following essential oils: rose, lavender, camphor, sage, rosemary, geranium, basil, cinnamon, clove, fennel, hyssop, jasmine, juniper, lemongrass, parsley, peppermint, and thyme[92].

- Avoid over-the-counter and prescription-only acne medications, including antibiotics, cortisone creams, and benzoyl peroxide. If you have severe acne please consult your OB-GYN before treating your skin with any medication.

- Avoid skin lightening products that may contain soy proteins which may disrupt hormonal balance in future mom and her developing baby.

- Avoid foaming cleansers and chemical-based body washes that contain sodium lauryl sulphate. Use organic cleansers or plain olive soaps to wash your face.

- Avoid using salicylic acid and aspiring masks as well as alpha- and beta-hydroxy acids in your cleansers, toners and moisturizers. Avoid acid-based home peels unless they are formulated with plant-derived glycolic acid.

- Avoid all skin care products that contain vitamin A, especially in form of retinol. Beta-carotene is proven to be safe, but studies are limited. As with many things in pregnancy, it is best to err on the side of caution.

- Avoid all skincare products that contain toxic ingredients, including preservatives. Check the Appendix A for the list of commonly used harmful skincare ingredients. Organic skin and body care products are the only way to go during pregnancy.

- Your skin is becoming very sensitive. Anything strongly scented can cause skin irritation. However, this is dangerous only if the scent is synthetic. Organic products may contain higher concentrations of essential oils so your skin needs some time to adjust.

Daily Skin Care Plan

Morning

- Remove the night treatment and refresh the skin with non-foaming or milky cleanser with gentle scrubbing particles.

- Refresh the skin with a gentle toner.

- Apply a topical treatment in a form of a serum or a light lotion.

- Apply a moisturizer that provides protection from sun and free radicals. A mineral foundation or lightweight mineral sunscreen, rain or shine, is the best way to avoid chloasma.

Evening

- Double-cleanse to remove makeup, sunscreen, and daily grime.

- Finish the cleansing with a toner to remove the cleanser residue and calm down your skin.

- Soothe and heal acne blemishes with a magnesium mask. To quickly dry out inflamed lesions and prepare your skin for a healthy night sleep apply a milk of magnesia for a few minutes.

- Apply a vitamin C powder directly on blemishes. To treat larger areas affected with acne mix with 1 scoop of philosophy Hope and a Prayer vitamin C with 2-3 drops of your favourite facial or body oil. Vitamin C will not dissolve completely. Please note: this concoction may sting.

- Delay and repair premature aging of eye area with intensive eye cream.
- Every other day: homemade scrub followed by a homemade mask to promote healing and fading of post-acne hyperpigmentation.
- Every week: a home microdermabrasion or a home peel.

Recommended Cleansers

$ Kiss My Face Olive Oil Soap
$ Weleda Calendula Baby Soap
$ Oliva Pure Olive Oil Soap
$ Weleda Iris Cleansing Lotion
$$ LUSH Baby Face Skin Cleanser
$$ Dr. Hauschka Cleansing Cream
$$$ Anne Marie Borlind ZZ Sensitive Cleansing Milk

Recommended Toners

$ Caudalie Grape Water
$ Avalon Organics Vitamin C Balancing Facial Toner
$$ Caudalie Beauty Elixir
$$ Origins Oil Refiner

Recommended Moisturizers/Sun Protection

$ Aubrey Organics Green Tea and Ginkgo SPF 15 Moisturiser
$ Trevarno Organic SPF 15 Day Cream
$$ Bare Escentuals i.d. bareMinerals Foundation SPF 15
$$ Aubrey Organics Sea Buckthorn with Ester-C Rejuvenating Antioxidant Serum
$$ Dr. Hauschka Sunscreen Lotion SPF 15 (for normal/dry skin)
$$ MD Formulations Total Protector 30
$$ Juice Beauty SPF 30 Tinted Moisturizer
$$$ Korres Watermelon Sunscreen Face Cream SPF 30
$$$ Jurlique Herbal Recovery Gel
$$$ Jane Iredale PurePressed Base SPF18
$$$ Patyka Organic Face Cream—Dry Skin

Recommended Topical Treatments

$ Eleusian Rose Hip Face Oil (for dry, dull skin)
$ Kalaya Emu Oil (for dryness, stretch marks)
$ Weleda Body Oil Sea Buckthorn (for stretch marks, great all over oil)
$$ LUSH Soft Coeur Massage Bar (for stretch marks)
$$ philosophy Prayer in a Bottle (directly on acne and hyperpigmentation)
$$$ Juice Beauty Antioxidant Serum (spots)

Recommended Eye Creams

$ Aubrey Organics Lumessence Rejuvenating Eye Crème
$ Avalon Organic Botanicals Vitamin C Revitalizing Eye Cream
$$ Juice Beauty Green Apple Nutrient Eye Cream
$$ Dr. Hauschka Daily Revitalizing Eye Cream

Baby Acne

Acne in newborns, or neonatal acne, is more common that we think. In fact, one in five newborns will have small, red bumps and pustules caused by temporary hormonal imbalances. Usually baby acne is scattered over the cheeks, forehead and sometimes even chest. There are no blackheads or whiteheads, and it's not harmful for the child. Baby acne typically appears at approximately 2 to 3 weeks of life. Baby boys are more commonly affected than girls.

Conventionally-thinking doctors would treat baby acne with topical antibiotics, benzoyl peroxide and even low concentration of tretinoin (Retin-A). These are hardly the substances you want near your precious little baby. Baby's skin is very thin and fragile, and its immune system will fully develop only by the age of nine months. Until that age, the child is more susceptible to infection and allergies because the skin is not yet able to defend itself against potential pathogens. That's why many topical treatments may cause allergic rash which could be even more harmful than baby acne. This is why many topical drugs, especially alcohol-based products, cannot be used on children under three years of age.

Always think about possible toxicity whenever you apply anything to a baby's skin. If you are concerned about treating your baby's acne with antibiotics or benzoyl peroxide talk to your doctor.

ACNE IN AGING SKIN

Are you suddenly dealing with the cosmetic double trouble of acne and wrinkles? You are not alone. The skin is one of the largest organs of the body, and it's one of the first to show the first signs of aging process and menopause. Estrogen fluctuations affect the cellular metabolism in skin, which leads to changes in the collagen and water content in the skin, along with dryness, atrophy, fine wrinkling, poor healing, and hot flashes. The skin starts lacking elasticity and strength, and wrinkles form. Contraceptive therapies and hormone treatments can also trigger or aggravate acne, especially during the perimenopausal period.

If you have to deal with acne that tarnishes your mature skin, you most probably have oily sensitive skin. Oily (or combination oily) skin is a mixed blessing. While women who had normal to dry skin in their 30s reach for anti-wrinkle creams in their 40s, you oily, taut skin resists aging more successfully. Since acne is no news to you, most likely you have an array of dark spots and freckles from previous acne outbreaks, sunbathing, and increased estrogen levels. Red or brown patches, broken facial capillaries

While dealing with acne and wrinkles, target the acne first. Anti-aging products may prevent and diminish wrinkles, but these may contain harsh ingredients, such as fruit acids, that can irritate your skin and worsen your acne by increasing burning and redness. Since the hormonal cause of acne in mature skin is rare, most often what you think is acne breakouts is in fact an allergic response to many skin care products. Sometimes red inflamed bumps are accompanied by redness, stinging, and burning.

Acne in aging skin requires gentler alternatives to zit zappers you used in your teenage years. In general, creamy cleansers, non-alcohol toners, and rich moisturizers work best for sensitive mature skin. If you have active acne breakouts, washing with salicylic-acid based cleansers to keep pores clean and using topical treatment only once a day will help calm down the skin. As soon as the inflammation is gone, switch back to your gentle, creamy cleansers and moisturizers.

General Guidelines for Aging Acne-Prone Skin

- Make sure you thoroughly remove makeup using double-cleanse technique and cleansers that do not contain alcohol or soap. Instead, choose milky cleansers that remove makeup without stripping your skin's natural oils. Look for ingredients such as aloe vera, green tea, calendula, chamomile, vitamin C. Avoid cold creams and cream cleansers.

- Use a toner with alpha-hydroxy acids every day to slough dead skin cells off the skin surface. Discontinue use if the toner stings or causes any other discomfort. Chamomile, aloe, cucumber, calendula and green tea added to a toner will provide an extra soothing and antioxidant effect.

- Every other day gently polish your skin with a non-scrubbing exfoliating cream or fluid that contains glycolic acid, botanical enzymes such as papain (papaya enzyme), bromelain (pineapple enzyme) to dissolve dead skin cells and help fade post-acne hyperpigmentation.

- Choose acne medications that do not contain benzoyl peroxide. Avoid drying serums and lotions that can exacerbate irritation and dryness. Choose natural-based acne medication that contains salicylic acid, tea tree oil or vitamin A.

- Wear a daily moisturizer rich in humectants (ingredients that hold moisture in your skin) such as hyaluronic acid, glycerin and sorbitol, and antioxidants such as vitamin C, green tea, tocopherol, grape seed extract, gingko biloba, Echinacea, and beta carotene. Pat your moisturizer with your fingertips—do not rub!—to avoid unnecessary stretching of the skin.

- Serums work perfectly for your skin because they contain active ingredients in higher concentration compared to regular moisturizers and night creams. Serums also penetrate better and stay on your skin longer. Costly as they are, serums usually last longer than moisturizers, too, because you only need a few drops to cover your face. You can also use serums sparingly around eyes but not too close to the lash line. At morning and night, use a serum or a lotion packed with botanical anti-aging ingredients such as caffeine from green tea, wild yam, pomegranate seed oil, niacinamide, superoxide dismutase, alpha lipoic acid, grape seed proanthocyanidins, hyaluronic acid, GABA (gamma aminobutyric acid), seaweed (algae), evening primrose oil, *Boswellia serrata*, and *Centella asiatica*.

- Regular moisturizing masks and at-home hydrating facials will help soothe redness and add moisture to your skin.

- If you have dark spots, apply topical skin lightening products after you have cleansed and toned your skin. Follow the topical product with your moisturizer and sunblock of choice. Begin to use skin whitening products on new and old dark spots and continue to use until the discoloration has completely disappeared.

- Vitamin C is a great ingredient that helps diminish pigmentation, wrinkles and acne. Choose a serum that contains freeze-dried vitamin C to normalize pigment cells, reduce acne inflammation and boost collagen production. You can also add powdered vitamin C to your moisturizers and sunblocks.

- Choose the sunscreen you will enjoy to wear. Since your skin is on the sensitive side, mineral sunscreens that contain titanium dioxide and zinc oxide are tolerated better.

- Mineral makeup is recommended if you are prone to acne. However, mineral powder foundations can accentuate fine lines and wrinkles due to their texture and a slight amount of shimmer in them. Instead of a powder, use fluid mineral makeup such as Jane Iredale Liquid Minerals.

- Take your daily dose of vitamins and antioxidants with additional alpha lipoic acid and omega 3 fatty acid supplements.

Top Five Things to Avoid

- Avoid abrasive scrubs that contain crushed seeds, sugar or salt. These can further irritate your skin adding to the problem.

- Never expose your skin to abrupt changes in temperatures, such as cold water splashes after cleansing or hot water compresses on acne.

- Don't rub your skin after shower or washing your face. Instead, pat your face dry with a separate face towel, and change it frequently.

- Don't use acne lotions and serums more often than once a day. If you absolutely must apply acne medication on the whole face, mix it in equal proportions with your regular moisturizer or anti-aging serum.

- Avoid products that contain ingredients most likely to cause allergic reaction. These usually are fragrances, color, penetration enhancers, and preservatives of all kinds. Make well-informed choices when buying skincare and choose anti-aging products that are as clean and "green" as possible.

Daily Skin Care Plan

Morning

- Remove the night treatment and refresh the skin with gentle milky cleanser with fruit acids or enzymes.

- Soothe and moisturize your skin with a toner.

- Apply a treatment of your choice: whitening, moisturizing, or wrinkle-relaxing serum.

- Top the treatment with a full-spectrum sunblock, mineral foundation or lightweight mineral sunscreen.

Evening

- Double-cleanse to remove makeup, sunscreen, and daily grime.

- Finish the cleansing with a toner to remove the cleanser residue and calm down your skin.

- Soothe and heal acne blemishes with a magnesium mask.

- Apply a concentrated serum of your choice or gentle acne medication.

- Apply a rich nighttime moisturizer that nourishes your skin while you sleep.

- Repair the delicate skin in the eye area with an intensive eye cream.

Recommended Cleansers

$ Avalon Organics Facial Cleansing Milk, Lavender
$ Weleda Iris Cleansing Lotion
$ Alba Botanica Sea Lettuce Cleansing Milk
$ Beauty Without Cruelty Facial Cleansing Milk, Extra Gentle
$$ MD Formulations Facial Cleanser—All Skin Types
$$ LUSH Baby Face Skin Cleanser
$$ Dr. Hauschka Cleansing Cream
$$ DHC Deep Cleansing Oil (for double-cleansing)
$$$ Suki Moisture Rich Face Cleanser
$$$ Dermalogica Precleanse (for double-cleansing)

Recommended Toners

$ Aubrey Organics Natural AHA Fruit Acids with Apricot Toning Moisturizer
$ Avalon Organics CoQ10 Perfecting Facial Toner
$ Caudalie Grape Water
$$ Kiss My Face Organics Balancing Act
$$ Rachel Perry Violet Rose Skin Toner
$$ derma e DMAE Alpha Lipoic C-Ester Firming Facial Toner
$$ Burt's Bees Carrot Seed Oil Complexion Mist for dry skin
$$$ Pangea Italian Green Mandarin with Sweet Lime
$$$ Caudalie Beauty Elixir

Recommended Moisturizers/Sun Protection

$ Beauty Without Cruelty Vitamin C, SPF 12 Facial Lotion wtih CoQ10
$$ Kiss My Face Organics Cell Mate 15, Facial Creme & Sunscreen SPF 15
$$ Dr. Hauschka Sunscreen Lotion SPF 15 (for normal/dry skin)
$$ MD Formulations Total Protector 30
$$ Zia Natural Skincare Daily Moisture Screen SPF 15
$$$ Korres Watermelon Sunscreen Face Cream SPF 30
$$$ Jane Iredale Liquid Minerals

Recommended Acne Treatments

$ Desert Essence Clear Skin Clear Conscience
$$ MD Formulations Vit A Plus Clearing Complex
$$ philosophy Prayer in a Bottle
$$$ Dr Brandt Poreless Gel
$$$ Kinerase Clear Skin Treatment Serum

Recommended Night Treatments

$$ Aubrey Organics Sea Buckthorn with Ester-C Rejuvenating Antioxidant Serum
$$ Primavera Ultra-Rich Energizing Seed Oil Capsules
$$ Philosophy When Hope Is Not Enough
$$ Suki Complexion Brightening Cream
$$$ REN Clean Skincare Repair Treatment
$$$ Cellex-C High Potency Serum
$$$ Dr. Hauschka Rhythmic Conditioner Sensitive
$$$ Jurlique Herbal Recovery Gel

$$$ Origins Plantidote Mega-Mushroom Face Serum
$$$ Givenchy No Surgetics Visible Resurfacing Serum

Recommended Eye Creams

$ Kiss My Face Organics Eyewitness, Eye Repair Creme
$ Burt's Bees Beeswax & Royal Jelly Eye Crème
$$ Jason Red Elements Lifting Eye Cream
$$ Anne Marie Borlind Eye Wrinkle Cream
$$ derma e Peptides Double Action Wrinkle Reverse Eye Creme
$$ Zia Natural Skincare Ultimate Eye Creme
$$$ Jurlique Eye Gel

Recommended Peels

$ Neutrogena Advanced Solutions Facial Peel
$$ MD Formulations Alpha Beta Daily Face Peel
$$ Juice Beauty Green Apple Peel—Full Strength
$$$ Kinerase Instant Radiance Facial Peel
$$$ Fresh Appleseed Resurfacing Kit

Maintaining Ageless Clear Skin

Coping with acne and wrinkles requires double effort, but over time, you'll be happy that your skin is on the oilier side. Oily/combination skin does require constant upkeep, but it also ages more slowly. You will develop wrinkles later, you are less prone to skin sagging, and although you might be prone to dark circles, your eye area remains youthful for much longer than in normal and dry skin types.

Botox, chemical peels, and microdermabrasion offer great results, but if you have oily skin the regular use of sunscreen, gentle skincare with anti-inflammatory and anti-oxidant products will also help stave off wrinkles just as effectively. However, if your skin bears the tell-tale signs of past acne damage, you may wish to explore cosmetic procedures. Intense Pulsed Light (IPL) therapy helps diminish brown spots, acne and wrinkles with practically no downtime. Salicylic and glycolic acid peels are also great for clearing acne, reducing brown spots and boosting collagen production. You may also use at-home natural glycolic peels listed above.

Your best bet for age-proofing your skin is a diet rich in natural antioxidants such as vitamin C, vitamin E, beta-carotene, lutein, lycopene, vitamin B2, coenzyme Q10, and cysteine (an amino acid). You may also want to enrich your diet with anti-oxidant herbs such as milk thistle, aloe vera, bilberry, ginkgo, grape seed and pine bark extracts. There are many anti-aging supplements available, from high-end, such as Dr. Weil Plantidote Mega-Mushroom Supplement or N.V. Perricone M.D. Skin & Total Body Nutritional Supplements. Regular stress relief and exercise routine helps tone both your skin and your body. And last but not least, practice rigorous sun protection and check all your suspicious moles and spots with your doctor.

BODY ACNE

In some people, acne problems are not confined to the face. No matter if it is caused by stress or hormonal fluctuations, acne knows no boundaries, and acne outbreaks on face or chest have the same origin as the facial ones. Occasional pimples can occur on all parts of your body, but sometimes acne outbreaks can become persistent. The neck, chest, back, shoulders and buttocks are the most common areas where acne can appear. Body skin is thicker and more resilient than facial skin, and acne tends to hang on for longer.

Body acne takes form of whiteheads, blackheads, pimples, pustules, and even cysts. Apart from hormonal shifts, stress and diet, body acne is often caused by irritation from mechanical friction on the skin. Bra and backpack straps, even itchy wool sweaters and annoying clothing labels can all cause irritation. Fitness clothing is also to blame. Tight-fitting tank tops and yoga pants, especially made of thick spandex, don't always allow for easy perspiration, causing your skin pores to swell and more prone to irritation and acne. Even poor-fitting panties can provoke acne on buttocks.

Treatments for body acne are pretty much the same as for facial acne, with two differences. First of all, body skin is more thick and resilient, which allows for using stronger lotions and potions. It also responds well to vigorous exfoliation but unlike face won't form dark spots just as easily. Second, body acne usually appears on areas that are hard to reach. While you can rub some salicylic acid lotion and even concealer on spots on your chest and shoulders, treating back acne (dubbed as "bacne") and buttocks often involves almost acrobatic contortions.

General Guidelines for Acne-Prone Body Skin

- Take a daily shower with a salicylic-acid-based shower gel. Wipe the area with a salicylic acid pad and follow with lightweight body moisturizer to protect the skin and promote healing.

- Avoid scrubbing acne-prone areas with washcloth or loofah. Instead, exfoliate using scrub with mild granules, and for a daily shower wash with your hands or at least a soft sponge that can be thoroughly rinsed off.

- Take a shower as soon as possible after physical activity. Don't shower with hot water that stimulates blood flow to the blemishes and make them more inflamed and swollen.

- Use a salicylic acid or tea tree oil spot treatment on acne pimples at night.

- Don't pick at your pimples: they will need more time to heal and will leave unsightly spots that tend to linger long after acne is gone.

- Don't be tempted to dry your acne in tanning salon or at the beach. Sun may actually trigger acne and increase your risk for skin cancer. If you must tan, cover areas affected by acne with lightweight sunblock. Tanning is a sure-fire way to dark post-acne spots. Luckily for you, they tend to vanish faster than on the face.

- Check your clothes for details that may increase friction and rethink your wardrobe for at least a few weeks until pimples are gone. Swap bras with scratchy lacy straps for attractive sport tanks and consider cotton underwear, as synthetic clothes are more likely to trap perspiration underneath and promote pimples.

Anti-Acne Body Treatment

Even with a twice-a-day shower and healthy habits such as blocking sun sometimes you may need a high performance special treatment, say, before an important event where you plan to wear a revealing evening dress or a beach date which is calling for that gorgeous bikini number. Here's an anti-acne body treatment that you can enjoy on a Friday night or Saturday morning once a week—or even every day, if you need results fast.

There are two ways to prep your skin for a "body facial"—a shower, if you are running short of time, or a relaxing bath if you have the whole evening ahead. For a shower, make sure to spend at least two minutes soaking in warm (not hot!) water using a salicylic-based shower gel. We tried and loved Zapzyt Acne Wash with Soothing Aloe & Chamomile and Lancome Body Delisse Immediate Soft Touch Moisturizing Body Wash. The latter is not the safest in terms of ingredients but it's a better choice for drier skin types. We don't recommend using popular Murad Acne Body Wash because it contains such ingredients as triclosan and hydrogen peroxide both of which are potentially toxic and have been shown to increase skin's sensitivity. In any case make sure not to use any of body washes on your face or hair.

For a relaxing antibacterial skin bath, dissolve 1 cup Epsom salts in warm water. Add 5 drops of chamomile oil, 5 drops of lemon oil (or ½ sliced lemon) and 1 cup of strongly brewed green tea. If you prefer a ready-made solution, Kneipp Thermal Spring Bath Salts with Lavender or Eucalyptus are great for acne-prone skin. Relax in the bath for at least 20 minutes with a cup of herbal tea to soothe jangled nerves.

Now it's time to exfoliate your body to get the most of the anti-acne mask we will apply later. Opt for a gentler scrub so you won't overstimulate your acne-prone areas. Choose a scrub that contains most of smallest possible microbeads. The texture should be creamy, not runny, and when you try the scrub on your hand, there should be many tiny particles left, not just a few large beads. If the scrub hurts your hand when you rub it in the store, it will be too harsh for your body acne.

The best way to get the scrub you like is to prepare it yourself. You will need 1 cup (200 ml) of body oil (any type by Ecco Bella, Dr. Hauschka, Alba Botanicals or Weleda) and about 1 cup of fine sea salt or brown sugar. Mix the salt/sugar and oil in a glass jar. You may add a drop or two of your favourite essential oil or chamomile and tea tree oil for added anti-acne benefits.

Apply the body scrub in circular motions starting at your legs and working upwards to stimulate blood circulation. Be extra gentle while exfoliating chest area and anywhere near inflamed pimples. If you rub too vigorously you risk rupturing the pimple and further irritating your skin. The right exfoliation should leave a light, temporarily redness caused by increased blood flow. Rinse the scrub and massage the remaining oil into your skin. Take another dip in your bath. It's now becoming more moisturizing as the oil accumulates on the surface.

The most important part of the anti-acne body treatment is the clay mask. To prepare a body mask, mix ½ cup of white or blue clay with ½ cup of strongly brewed green tea and 2 tsp of honey. Stir thoroughly so there are no lumps. Apply the mask generously over the areas affected by acne and leave to dry. You may also use any of the recommended masks for teenage skin.

When the mask dries, rinse it off and pat the skin dry with a clean towel. Apply a topical treatment with tea tree oil, salicylic acid (not if you are pregnant!) or for emergency, vitamin C powder (philosophy Hope and a Prayer) mixed with 3-5 drops of rose hip or evening primrose oil applied directly on pimples. Beware: it may sting. Finish the "body facial" with a lightweight moisturizer such as Avalon Organics Lavender Therapeutic Hand & Body Lotion, Jason Natural Cosmetics Aloe Vera 70% All-Over Body Lotion or Kiss My Face Oil Free Moisturizer with NaPCA. If you plan to wear a low-cut or sleeveless dress, you may wish to dust the acne breakouts with a mineral foundation. Powder or cream bronzer may play down dark post-acne spots, but anything shimmery will instantly accentuate any skin roughness or prominent zits.

Spa Procedures for Body Acne

Body scrubs

Spa body scrubs are in principle the same as face scrubs—but much more self-indulgent. During the procedure the therapist massages the scrub onto the body starting with legs, while the rest of your body relaxes under the warm blanket or a cotton sheet. Most spa-quality body scrubs are made with sea salts or brown sugar, both of which are great for acne-prone skin. Essential oils, floral essences, clays and mud, even red wine and fruit pulp all help refresh and renew the skin. The scrub is then removed with hot steamed towels or shower. Sometimes the body scrub is followed with sunless tanning session. Please note that body scrubs and self-tanners are not recommended if you are pregnant or nursing.

Body wraps

Before the body wrap, an aesthetician would perform a dry brushing or a full body exfoliation so that your skin would be able to perspire better. Then the body is painted with mud, clay or various masks—sometimes even chocolate!—depending on the spa. Then your body is wrapped in metallic foil or plastic, sometimes topped with heated blankets to stimulate the perspiration and to help flush toxins from the skin. After you spend from 30 minutes to an hour in this decadent cocoon, an herbal, mineral bath, hot steamed towel massage or Vichy shower treatment follows. Please note that you would be provided with disposable panties before the procedure so your precious lacy underwear won't be ruined.

Thalassotherapy

This spa procedure was developed in France in the 19th century. Thalassotherapy is based on use of sea water which is rich in magnesium, potassium, and calcium sulphate, which are particularly beneficial for body acne. Various types of seaweed are well known for their antibiotic, antibacterial and antiviral properties. During thalassotherapy, your body is showered with warmed seawater, then covered with marine mud, algae or sea salt mask and then wrapped in seaweed previously soaked in sea water. After you linger in this warm wrap—feeling pretty much like a delicious sushi roll—the concoction is rinsed off in with a hydrotherapeutic or Vichy shower. Again, this treatment may not be suitable if you are pregnant or nursing.

Hydrotherapy

This is basically a relaxing soak in a therapeutic hot tub with herbal concoctions, salts, and essential oils that help you sweat out toxins and relax. Hydrotherapy may follow the body wrap and body scrub. Another type of hydrotherapy is the Vichy shower that consists of a row of shower heads which pour water while you lay on a massage table.

Balneotherapy

This procedure is basically bathing in thermal water baths and pools. Balneotherapy was practiced by ancient Greeks and Romans, and the first spas in the 1800s in Europe were built on thermal springs. Many mineral baths contain sulfur which is great for treating and preventing acne, as well as dermatitis and rosacea. Among the most popular balneological centers with sulphur-rich water are Carlsbad and Marienbad in Germany, luxurious Bagni di Pisa in Italy, Balneario de Blancafort in Spain, Altiplano Hot Springs in Chile and Sycamore Mineral Springs Resort in San Luis Obispo, California. Other famous thermal water destinations include Budapest in Hungary and Tuscany in Italy.

CONCLUSION

Red, inflamed acne zits. Benzoyl Peroxide. New inflammation. Stress. Anxiety. More zits, more harsh measures that ruin your skin and leave you desperate. We all have been through this watching as acne is tarnishing our looks and crippling our spirits.

Here, now, you have everything you need to end this vicious circle. Just like allergy sufferers carefully avoid any substances that could trigger their allergies, you can avoid anything that may provoke your acne. With this complete collection of all-natural organic solutions for your acne problems, you have learned how to adjust your diet, practice stress relief and choose the right natural skincare suitable for your skin type. These techniques are easy and affordable, and they make a great difference to your skin and body at whole. Remarkably down-to-earth as they seem, these small changes and simple techniques are extremely effective against your acne.

It's easier said than done, but don't try to get caught in the magical bullet expectation loop. Unrealistic expectations—looking for fast results with minimal effort—lead to frustration and more stress. There are no miracles when you deal with your skin, and don't get fooled by anyone who promises you clear skin in three days. Don't feel like you are doomed with acne for life, either. Stay in control of your diet and skincare routine and don't get upset if you cannot put into practice all the new things at once. It's also important not to compare yourself to the models on magazine pages. For every photo taken there are hours of airbrush makeup application and Photoshop retouching. Instead of getting discouraged by all those teenage silky-faced sirens in fashion magazines take a constructive approach: make an extra-cleansing facial mask, meditate, and eat an apple or two.

Most of all, it's our greatest hope that your awareness of your skin's health has reached new heights. Letting go of old practices of dealing with acne will make a great impact on your skin's health for many years to come. Remember that you are now armed with knowledge to make informed choices in your skincare and diet. Going green in your beauty habits may not be as easy as it seems, but very soon you will be rewarded with glowing and healthy—not just healthy-looking—acne-free complexion.

APPENDIX A

LIST OF COMMONLY USED HARMFUL SKINCARE INGREDIENTS*

Toxic Ingredients

Alcohol Denat (SD Alcohol 40-B)—classified as toxic, reproductive/developmental toxicity

Benzyl Alcohol—classified as toxic, may cause allergies and sensitization

Benzophenone-3 (oxybenzone)—classified as toxic, estrogenic chemicals and endocrine disruptor

Ceteareth-20—unsafe for use in cosmetics, penetration enhancer

Cocamide DEA—cancer hazard, immune system toxicant

Cocamide MEA—cancer hazard, immune system toxicant

Dimethyl MEA (monoethanolamine)—cancer hazard, immune system toxicant

Diazolidinyl Urea—classified as toxic, immune system toxicant

Hydrogen Peroxide—classified as toxic, cancer hazard, immune system toxicant

Iodopropynyl Butylcarbamate—classified as toxic, unsafe for use in cosmetics, reproductive toxicant

Imidazolidinyl Urea—classified as toxic, immune system toxicant

Isobutylparaben—classified as toxic, estrogenic chemical, endocrine disruptor

Isopropyl Alcohol (SD-40)—classified as toxic, eye, skin, or lungs irritant

Germaben (paraben)—classified as toxic, estrogenic chemical, endocrine disruptor

Methylparaben—classified as toxic, estrogenic chemical, endocrine disruptor

PEG-6, PEG-32—unsafe for use in cosmetics

PEG-80 Sorbitan Laurate—classified as toxic, immune system toxicant

Methylisothiazolinone—immune system toxicant

Octyl Methoxy-Cinnamate—estrogenic chemical, endocrine disruptor

Phenoxyethanol—classified as toxic, reproductive toxicant, eye, skin, or lungs irritant

Propylene Glycol—immune system toxicant, penetration enhancer

Propylparaben—classified as toxic, estrogenic chemical, endocrine disruptor
Quaternium-15—classified as toxic, immune system toxicant
Polyquaternium-10—may contain harmful impurities
Polysorbate-20—classified as toxic, may cause allergies and sensitization
Polyethylene—cancer hazard, may cause allergies, sensitization
Sodium Metabisulfite (sulfite)—classified as toxic, immune system toxicant
Sodium Dehydroacetate—classified as toxic
Triclosan—classified as toxic, immune system toxicant, eye, skin, or lungs irritant
Triethanolamine—cancer hazard, safety limits on use, immune system toxicant, skin irritant

Skin Irritants

Aminomethyl Propanol
Benzophenone-4
Cocamidopropyl Betaine
Disodium EDTA
DMDM Hydantoin
Methylisothiazolinone
Sodium Laureth Sulfate
Tetrasodium EDTA
Urea
Potassium Hydrochloride

Not Yet Tested for Safety

Butylene Glycol
Caprilyc/capric triglyceride
Cyclopentasiloxane
Dimethicone
Dipotassium Glycyrrhizate
Disodium Lauroamphodiacetate
Ethoxydiglycol
Hexyldecanol
Hydroxypropyl Cyclodextrin
Isododecane Isohexadecane
Lauramide MEA (monoethanolamine)
Methyl Gluceth-20
Neopentyl Glycol Dicaprate

Neopentyl Glycol Diisostearate
PEG-100 Stearate
PEG-120 Methyl Glucose Dioleate
Pentaethythrityl Tetraoctanoate
Pentylene Glycol
Petrolatum
PPG-12/SMDI Copolymer
Sodium Lauroamphoacetate
Sodium Trideceth Sulfate
Sodium Hydroxide
TEA Cocoyl Alaninate
Tributyl Citrate

* Based on EWG SkinDeep Report and ingredients lists of more than 100 commonly available beauty products

Top 20 Brands of Concern

Skin Deep's safety assessment ratings provide a measure of potential health concerns linked to ingredients used in popular health and beauty brands. (In brackets—the manufacturer of the brand).

1. Dark & Lovely (L'Oréal)
2. Chanel (Chanel)
3. Lierac (ALES Group USA)
4. Clarins (Clarins Paris)
5. Banana Boat (Playtex Products)
6. Te Tao (Kuan Ltd.)
7. Back to Basics (Graham Webb International)
8. Ultima II (Revlon)
9. Estée Lauder (Estée Lauder)
10. Fresh (Fresh)
11. Sally Hansen (Del Laboratories, Inc.)
12. B. Kamins (Kamins Dermatologics)
13. Murad (Murad)
14. Revlon (Revlon)
15. Clairol (Procter & Gamble)
16. Freeman (pH Beauty Labs)
17. Elizabeth Arden (Elizabeth Arden)

18. Gillette (Procter & Gamble)
19. Artec (ARTec Systems Group)
20. Color Me Beautiful (Color Me Beautiful)

APPENDIX B

WHERE TO CHECK FOR INGREDIENT SAFETY

Environmental Working Group

ewg.org/reports/skindeep2

Here you can browse your favourite skincare, hair and body products as well as nail care, baby products, and fragrances. The easy-to-use database allows searching for specific ingredients and helps create beauty shopping lists based on your preferences.

Hazardous Substances Data Bank

toxnet.nlm.nih.gov/

Databases on toxicology, hazardous chemicals, environmental health, and toxic releases. Search by ingredient to check the latest research.

U.S. Environment Protection Agency

epa.gov/iris/index.html

IRIS Database for Risk Assessment lists various substances found in the environment and human health effects that may result from exposure to them. Search the database by keyword or list of substances.

Household Products Database

householdproducts.nlm.nih.gov

Learn more about what's under your kitchen sink, in your garage, in your bathroom, and on the shelves in your laundry room. Search by ingredient and product for potential health effects, about safety and handling recommendations.

Ingredients Prohibited and Restricted by FDA Regulations

cfsan.fda.gov/~dms/cos-210.html

The list of chemical substances prohibited for use in cosmetics for safety concerns or environmental factors. "Cosmetic ingredients are not subject to FDA premarket approval authority," the list warns.

APPENDIX C

WHERE TO BUY ACNE SKIN CARE PRODUCTS

Anne Marie Borlind: better spa and salons, online at borlind.com, drugstore.com, naturalskinandhair.com

Anthony Logistics: better spa and salons, online at sephora.com

Aveda: Aveda stores worldwide, online at aveda.com

Aveeno: most supermarket and drugstore chains worldwide, online at drugstore.com

Aubrey Organics: health food stores, online at aubrey-organics.com, theremustbeabetterway.co.uk, amazon.com

Australian Organics: online at australianorganics.net, drugstore.com

Bare Escentuals: in Sephora stores and online, Nordstrom, Ulta, online at bareescentuals.com, amazon.com.

Beauty Without Cruelty: at health food stores, online at beautywithoutcruelty.com, drugstore.com, mothernature.com

Benefit: in Sephora stores and online, Benefit boutiques, The Bay (Canada), Galeries Lafayette (France), Bloomingdale's (USA), online at benefit.com

Biotherm: in selected department stores, online at benefit-us.com, sephora.com

Boscia: in Sephora stores and online

Burt's Bees: in better health food stores, online at burtsbees.com, amazon.com, drugstore.com

Caudalie: in selected department stores, Sephora stores and online, better pharmacies (France)

D'Arcy: online at darcyskincare.com

Derma-E—in health food stores, Wal-Mart (Canada), online at dermae.net, drugstore.com, shopping.com

Dermalogica: in Dermalogica salons worldwide, online at amazon.com, hqhair.com

Desert Essence: health food stores, online at desertessence.com

DHC Skincare: online at dhccare.com, Marukai Pacific Market Store (Gardena, CA, USA)

Dr. Hauschka: in better salons and spas, online at drhauschka.com, saffronerouge.com, eBay, amazon.com

Ecco Bella: in better salons and health stores, online at eccobella.com

Eleusian: online at eleusian.com.au

Emerita: online at emerita.com, drugstore.com

Givenchy: Saks (USA), Harrods (UK), Holt Renfrew (Canada), Sephora stores and online

Fresh: Sephora stores and online

Jason: health food stores, online at jason-natural.com

Jane Iredale: better salons, online at janeiredale.com, skinstore.com

Juice Beauty: in Sephora stores and online

Jurlique: better spa and salons, online at saffronrouge.com, eSkinStore.com

Kalaya: health stores, online at kalayacreations.com

Kinerase—in Sephora stores and online

Kiss My Face: health stores, online at drugstore.com

Korres: in Sephora stores and online

La Fleur Organique: Walgreens (USA), online at lafleurorganique.com

Living Nature: health stores, online at livingnature.com

LUSH: in LUSH stores worldwide, online at lush.com

MD Skincare: better salons and spa, in Sephora stores and online

Miessence: better salons and spa, online at miessenceproducts.com, theremustbeabetterway.co.uk, chooseorganics.com

Neutrogena: most supermarket and drugstore chains worldwide, online at drugstore.com

N.V.Perricone: online at nvperriconemd.com, Sephora.com, amazon.com

Origins: Bloomingdales, Macy's (USA), The Bay (Canada), Les Galeries Lafayette Haussmann (France), Harrods, Selfridges, John Lewis (UK), online at origins.com

Pangea: online at pangeaorganics.com, saffronrouge.com

Patyka: online at lusciouscargo.com, aedes.com

Philosophy: department stores worldwide, online at amazon.com, beauty.com, sephora.com

Primavera: online at primavera.co.uk, saffronrouge.com, holisticbeauty.net

Rachel Perry: health stores and beauty salons, online at rachelperry.net, drugstore.com

REN Clean Skincare: Space NK Apothecary (UK), online at renskincare.com

Suki Pure Skin Care: online at sukisnaturals.com

Tend Skin: better salons and beauty spas, online at sephora.com, folica.com

Thayer's: Vitamin Shoppe (USA), other better health food and beauty locations, online at thayers.com

The Body Shop: store locations worldwide, online at thebodyshop.com

Trevarno: online at trevarnoskincare.co.uk, theremustbeabetterway.co.uk

Weleda: better salons and health food stores, online at weleda.com (site in German), usa-weleda.com, and drugstore.com

ZAPZYT: Rite-Aid, Ulta, Walgreens, Wal-Mart and other pharmacies (USA), online at drugstore.com

Zia Natural Skincare: Vitamin Shoppe, other better health food stores in the USA, online at drugstore.com

Zirh: Bloomingdales, Barneys, Saks Fifth Ave (USA), Holt Renfrew, Shoppers Drug Mart (Canada), Harrods, Selfridges, House of Fraser (UK), online at zirh.com, amazon.com, Sephora.com

REFERENCES

1. Brajac I, Bilic-Zulle L, Tkalcic M, Loncarek K, Gruber F. Acne vulgaris: myths and misconceptions among patients and family physicians. *Patient Education Counselor.* 2004 Jul; 54(1):21-5.

2. van der Meeren HL, van der Schaar WW, van den Hurk CM. The psychological impact of severe acne. *Cutis: cutaneous medicine for the practitioner.* 1985 Jul; 36(1):84-6.

3. Minciullo PL, Patafi M, Giannetto L, Ferlazzo B, Trombetta D, Saija A, Gangemi S. Allergic contact angioedema to benzoyl peroxide. *Journal of Clinical Pharmacy and Therapeutics.* 2006 Aug; 31(4):385-7

4. Slaga, T.J et al. Skin Tumor-Promoting Activity of Benzoyl Peroxide, a Widely Used Free Radical-Generating Compound. *Science.*28/8/81. Vol. 213, 1023-1024.

5. Mathur S, Kaur P, Sharma M, Katyal A, Singh B, Tiwari M, Chandra R. The treatment of skin carcinoma, induced by UV B radiation, using 1-oxo-5beta, 6beta-epoxy-witha-2-enolide, isolated from the roots of *Withania Somnifera*, in a rat model. *Phytomedicine.* 2004 Jul; 11(5):452-60.

6. Mancuso M, Pazzaglia S, Tanori M, Rebessi S, Di Majo V, Covelli V, Saran A. Only a subset of 12-O-tetradecanoylphorbol-13-acetate-promoted mouse skin papillomas is promotable by benzoyl peroxide. *Mutations Research.* 2004 Apr 14; 548(1-2):35-45.

7. Qiu C, Fu F, Gao Q, Wang C, Wen Y. The function of benzoyl peroxide in the induction of Syrian golden hamster tongue carcinoma by chemical carcinogen. Article in Chinese. *Hua Xi Kou Qiang Yi Xue Za Zhi.* 2000 Oct; 18(5):291-3.

8. Food and Drug Administration. Topical Drug Products Containing Benzoyl Peroxide; Required Labeling. Federal Register. 1995, February 17. Volume 60, No. 33: 9554-9556.

9. Opinion of The Scientific Committee on Cosmetic Products and Non-Food Products Intended for Consumers. Opinion on the use of Benzoyl Peroxide (BPO) Hydroquinone (HQ), Hydroquinone Methylether (MEHQ) in artificial nail systems adopted by the SCCNFP during the 20th plenary meeting of 04 June 2002. *EUROPA*, European Commission, DG Health and Consumer Protection, Public Health: ec.europa.eu/health

10. Burkman R, Schlesselman JJ, Zieman M. Safety concerns and health benefits associated with oral contraception. *American Journal of Obstetrics and Gynecology*. 2004; 190(4 Suppl): S5-22.

11. Ian S Fraser. Forty years of combined oral contraception: the evolution of a revolution. *The Medical Journal of Australia*. 2000; 173: 541-544.

12. Nouri K, Ballard CJ. Laser therapy for acne. *Clinics in Dermatology*. 2006 Jan-Feb; 24(1):26-32.

13. Hongcharu W, Taylor CR, Chang Y, Aghassi D, Suthamjariya K, Anderson RR. Topical ALA-photodynamic therapy for the treatment of acne vulgaris. *The Journal of Investigative Dermatology*. 2000 Aug; 115(2):183-92.

14. Kligman, D; Kligman, A.M. Salicylic Acid Peels for the Treatment of Photoaging. *Dermatologic Surgery*. 1998, March. Vol. 24, No. 3, Pages 325-328.

15. Chivot M. Retinoid therapy for acne. A comparative review. *American Journal of Clinical Dermatology*. 2005;6(1):13-9.

16. El-Akawi Z, Abdel-Latif N, Abdul-Razzak K. Does the plasma level of vitamins A and E affect acne condition? *Clinical and Experimental Dermatology*. 2006 May; 31 (3):430-4.

17. Sherertz EF. Acneiform eruption due to "megadose" vitamins B6 and B12. *Cutis; cutaneous medicine for the practitioner*. 1991 Aug; 48(2):119-20.

18. Keller, K.L., M.D.; Fenske, N.A. Uses of Vitamins A, C, and E and Related Compounds in Dermatology: A Review. *Journal of the American Academy of Dermatology*. 1998 October: 611-625.

19. Ayres S Jr, Mihan R, Scribner MD. Synergism of vitamins A and E with dermatologic applications. *Cutis; cutaneous medicine for the practitioner.* 1979 May;23 (5):600-3, 689-90.

20. Dreno B, Foulc P, Reynaud A, Moyse D, Habert H, Richet H. Effect of zinc gluconate on propionibacterium acnes resistance to erythromycin in patients with inflammatory acne: in vitro and in vivo study. *European Journal of Dermatology.* 2005 May-Jun; 15(3):152-5.

21. Stephan F, Revuz J. Zinc salts in dermatology. *Annales de Dermatologie et de Venereologie.* 2004 May; 131 (5):455-60.

22. Letawe C, Boone M, Pierard GE. Digital image analysis of the effect of topically applied linoleic acid on acne microcomedones. *Clinical and Experimental Dermatology.* 1998 Mar; 23 (2):56-8.

23. Berbis P, Hesse S, Privat Y. Essential fatty acids and the skin. *Allergie et Immunologie* (Paris). 1990 Jun; 22 (6):225-31.

24. Eby GA, Eby KL. Rapid recovery from major depression using magnesium treatment. *Medical Hypotheses.* 2006; 67 (2):362-70.

25. U.S. Food and Drug Administration, Center for Food Safety and Applied Nutrition *Dietary Supplement Health and Education Act of 1994.* U.S. Department of Health and Human Services. December 1, 1995.

26. Duker EM, Kopanski L, Jarry H, Wuttke W. Effects of extracts from Cimicifuga racemosa on gonadotropin release in menopausal women and ovariectomized rats. *Planta Med* 1991; 57:420-4.

27. Jiang C, Agarwal R, Lu J. Anti-angiogenic potential of a cancer chemopreventive flavonoid antioxidant, Silymarin: inhibition of key attributes of vascular endothelial cells and angiogenic cytokine secretion by cancer epithelial cells. *Biochemical and Biophysical Research Communications.* 2000; 276: 371-378.

28. McKenna DJ, Jones K, Humphrey S, Hughes K. Black cohosh: efficacy, safety, and use in clinical and preclinical applications. *Alternative Therapies in Health and Medicine.* 2001; 7:93-100.

29. Akamatsu H, Asada Y, Horio T. Effect of keigai-rengyo-to, a Japanese Kampo medicine, on neutrophil functions: a possible mechanism of action of keigai-rengyo-to in acne. *The Journal of International Medical Research.* 1997; 25:255-265.

30. Paranjpe, P., Kulkarni, P.H. Comparative efficacy of four Ayurvedic formulations in the treatment of acne vulgaris: a double-blind randomized placebo-controlled clinical evaluation. *The Journal of Ethnopharmacology.* 1995 Dec 15; 49(3):127-32.

31. Cordain L. Implications for the role of diet in acne. *Seminars in Cutaneous Medicine and Surgery.* 2005 Jun; 24(2):84-91.

32. Green J, Sinclair RD. Perceptions of acne vulgaris in final year medical student written examination answers. *The Australasian Journal of Dermatology.* 2001 May; 42(2):98-101.

33. Wolf R, Matz H, Orion E. Acne and diet. *Clinical Dermatology.* 2004 Sep-Oct; 22(5):387-93.

34. Fulton JE Jr, Plewig G, Kligman AM. Effect of chocolate on acne vulgaris. *JAMA.* 1969 Dec 15; 210(11):2071-4.

35. Giugliano D, Ceriello A, Esposito K. The effects of diet on inflammation: emphasis on the metabolic syndrome. *Journal of American College of Cardiology.* 2006 Aug 15; 48(4):677-85.

36. Sanchez, A, et al. Role of sugar in human neurophilic phagocytosis. *The American Journal of Clinical Nutrition.* 1973; 26: 1180-4

37. Bunselmeyer B. Probiotics and prebiotics for the prevention and treatment of atopic eczema. *Der Hautarzt: Zeitschrift fur Dermatologie, Venerologie und verwandte Gebiete.* 2005 October 21.

38. Black PH. Central nervous system-immune system interactions: psycho-neuroendocrinology of stress and its immune consequences. *Antimicrobial Agents and Chemotherapy.* 1994 Jan; 38 (1):1-6.

39. Thiboutot D. Acne: hormonal concepts and therapy. *Clinics in Dermatology.* 2004 Sep-Oct; 22(5):419-28.

40. Lucky AW. Quantitative documentation of a premenstrual flare of facial acne in adult women. *Archives of Dermatology.* 2004 Apr; 140(4):423-4.

41. Stoll S, Shalita AR, Webster GF, Kaplan R, Danesh S, Penstein A. The effect of the menstrual cycle on acne. *Journal of American Academy of Dermatology.* 2001 Dec; 45(6):957-60.

42. Faure M. Acne and hormones. *La Revue du Praticien.* 2002 Apr 15; 52 (8):850-3.

43. Khan MZ, Naeem A, Mufti KA. Prevalence of mental health problems in acne patients. *Journal of Ayub Medical College, Abbottabad: JAMC.* 2001 Oct-Dec; 13(4):7-8.

44. Cunliffe WJ. Acne and unemployment. *British Journal of Dermatology.* 1986 Sep 115(3):386.

45. Gupta MA, Gupta AK. Depression and suicidal ideation in dermatology patients with acne, alopecia areata, atopic dermatitis and psoriasis. *British Journal of Dermatology.* 1998 Nov; 139(5): 846-50.

46. Fried RG. Nonpharmacologic treatments in psychodermatology. *Dermatologic Clinics.* 2002 Jan; 20 (1):177-85.

47. Office of Radiation and Indoor Air (6604J). The Inside Story: A Guide to Indoor Air Quality. *U.S. Environmental Protection Agency and the United States Consumer Product Safety Commission.*1995, April. EPA Document # 402-K-93-007.

48. Gonzalez H, Farbrot A, Larko O, Wennberg AM. Percutaneous absorption of the sunscreen benzophenone-3 after repeated whole-body applications, with and without ultraviolet irradiation. *British Journal of Dermatology.* 2006 Feb; 154(2):337-40.

49. Korinth G, Weiss T, Angerer J, Drexler H. Dermal absorption of aromatic amines in workers with different skin lesions: a report on 4 cases. *Journal of Occupational Medical Toxicology.* 2006 Jul 19; 1(1):17.

50. Fulton JE Jr, Pay SR, Fulton JE 3rd. Comedogenicity of current therapeutic products, cosmetics, and ingredients in the rabbit ear. *Journal of the American Academy of Dermatology.* 1984 Jan; 10(1):96-105.

51. Topping DC, Bernard LG, O'Donoghue JL, English JC. Hydroquinone: Acute and subchronic toxicity studies with emphasis on neurobehavioral and nephrotoxic effects. *Food and Chemical Toxicology*. August 22, 2006.

978-0-595-42460-3
0-595-42460-0